HopePMDD

ISBN: 9798877567283

This book is dedicated to my wife.
Without her, this book would not be possible.

Contents

Introduction

Those who live with PMDD can suffer immensely, and the symptoms can ruin relationships, dreams, and aspirations. Living alongside someone with PMDD has been a life changing experience for me. Watching the development, fluctuations and influence of PMDD in my wife over 20 years has been a heartbreaking but fascinating journey.

Only those who have PMDD or lived alongside someone with the condition will know what a surreal experience it can be. In a bizarre, but predictable fashion, every month, those with PMDD can undergo a sudden unnerving change in disposition. For many, it's a cataclysmic bomb of anxiety, anger, depression and fatigue; PMDD is dragging her through hell, and you are coming along for the trip.

In many ways, this book is a letter to my younger self of things I wish I had known earlier on. There are many ways I would have acted differently had I understood the condition better. I wonder how many broken relationships could have been saved if PMDD had been understood. In a survey by the International Association for Premenstrual Disorders, *over half* of those with PMDD felt they lost a partner because of it.

Whilst this book is primarily for partners, I hope it will also be useful for others, including parents, friends and family members. To find some meaningful commentary on PMDD, I have also tried to draw from other people's experiences to ensure what I write is broadly representative of other people's PMDD experience.

Although I may refer to those who have PMDD as women in this book, I recognise that PMDD can be experienced by anyone who has a menstrual cycle, regardless of how they self-identify. Everything written in this book has been read by my wife, and I have her explicit permission to share what is written. At times I write with a degree of humour – I want to make it clear in advance that the humour is there to make such a weighty subject more palatable, not as a matter of levity on a serious condition.

I'd like to thank Chelsea @PMDDmemes on Instagram for allowing use of the PMDD memes you see scattered in the book. I would also like to thank those who read and provided feedback on the book's content or gave permission for me to use their words. Thanks Sophie at Durham University and to those at the International Association for Premenstrual Disorders (IAPMD) including Laura, Kelly, Marybeth and Sheila, who provide a lifeline for those who have PMDD. A special shout out to Sandi MacDonald, co-founder of IAPMD whose relentless perseverance and personal sacrifices for the PMDD community is super-human. Thank you also to my daughter Beth for the design work. Obviously, most of all, a big thanks to my wife Jude who is an inspiration to me in her strength, integrity and her unconditional compassion for every being under the sun, except for spiders.

1

UNDERSTANDING PMDD

What is PMDD?

Throughout a woman's life she will have approximately 480 periods. If PMDD symptoms last for one week (when quite often they last longer), that equates to more than nine years of PMDDing. That is a fair chunk of someone's life to feel awful.

PMDD is a relatively newly recognised condition in the medical world, having been added to the DSM-5[1] in 2013 and becoming an official worldwide diagnosis in January 2022 when its entry in the ICD-11[2] went live. You would think that being recognised officially by experts a lot of people would know about it. But its status is generally under-recognised, under-diagnosed, under-supported and misunderstood. While some medical professionals have a thorough understanding of PMDD, many have never heard of it!

So, what is it? Scientists say that Premenstrual Dysphoric Disorder (PMDD) is *"a condition that is an unholy hell of anguish, despair, and torment."* Oh, sorry, that's not *exactly* what scientists say. Scientists say that 'Premenstrual Dysphoric Disorder (PMDD) is a cyclical, hormone-based mood disorder with symptoms arising during the premenstrual, or luteal, phase of the menstrual cycle and subsiding within a few days of menstruation."

I like to describe PMDD as a *hypersensitivity to hormonal fluctuations*, an exaggerated or pathological response by the brain to the normal ebb and flow of the sex hormones.

---

[1] Diagnostic and Statistical Manual of Mental Disorders.

[2] The ICD-11 is produced by the World Health Organisation and catalogues known human diseases, medical conditions and mental health disorders and is used for tracking illnesses and as a global health categorization tool.

Most women will experience Premenstrual Symptoms (PMS), which can normally occur just before their period. PMS is NOT PMDD.

PMS is common. Some studies show that up to 70% of women will experience symptoms. Symptoms of Premenstrual Syndrome include: [3]

- mood swings
- feeling upset, anxious, or irritable
- tiredness or trouble sleeping
- bloating or stomach pain
- breast tenderness
- headaches
- spotty skin or greasy hair
- changes in appetite and sexual drive

PMS can be mild, moderate, or severe, but with PMDD, it's like the symptoms of PMS got *way* out of control. Instead of impacting or *influencing* someone's life, the symptoms start to run rampant and attempt to *dominate* that person's life (and subsequently those around the person). What really makes the difference between PMDD and PMS is the **severity of the symptoms** and how much it **impacts their life**. It is hard to communicate to people just **how bad** it can be.

Everyone gets headaches from time to time, perhaps if you are tired, dehydrated, or have a cold, but for the most part, with some water, sleep, or painkillers, people can go about their lives. Migraines are a brain explosion that can make people want to sit and cry in a dark room.

Headaches aren't migraines, and PMS isn't PMDD.

This is a barrier for people to understand. It is like a mental brick wall. You might try to explain to someone about PMDD and receive naive replies like ... "Yeah, my partner gets a bit moody before her period." "All women suffer

---

[3] https://www.mind.org.uk/information-support/types-of-mental-health-problems/premenstrual-dysphoric-disorder-pmdd/about-pmdd/

a bit, don't they?" "Maybe she doesn't cope as well as other women?" "It's all in her head." "She just needs to take control." "I have some essential oils that might cure her."

No.
You. Do. Not. Understand.

The severity of PMDD is difficult for others to understand because words like 'pain, anxiety, suffering, and depression' are all so subjective and can mean something different to each person, often based on their own personal experience. As a dentist I am fully versed in the spectrum of experiences that people can experience under the one-word umbrella of 'pain'; from the mild sharp transient sensitivity experienced during ice cream to the raging, overwhelming, head-splitting pain of an acute dental abscess. One person's pain is not another's and so it is with describing PMDD.

If PMS is an inconvenient spot of rain on a Sunday afternoon, then PMDD is a biblical-scale, force 5 hurricane. If PMS is a loving poodle, then PMDD is a starved rottweiler. It's the perfect storm of physiology and psychology (so don't let yourself get confused); they are not the same, and they deserve to be differentiated.

PMDD is also a spectrum disorder. That means that one person's symptoms might not be as extreme or intense as another's, or it might mean that they experience different predominant symptoms, e.g. in the luteal phase, for some, rage is the overbearing symptom, whereas for others it might be depression, anxiety or fatigue.

Whether symptoms are mild, moderate or severe they are at a level that interferes with daily life during the luteal phase. The fun thing? They can change over time or even month to month. I heard one partner call it 'the magical menstrual tour' - you never know what to expect!

PMDD sufferers often experience profound mood swings that bring unpredictability to life. "Mood swings" are one of those broad terms that people take and relate to their own experiences. That happens a lot, right?

You share your own experience with someone, and instead of listening or trying to understand further, the person immediately blurts out an experience that they had that they feel is similar. It's a bit like watching an episode of Baywatch and thinking you know what it's like to live in California.

One person's "mood swings" are not another's. When people say "mood swings," I normally think of the playground swings that swing from the centre in one direction at around 30 to 40 degrees. They are fun and enjoyable. If you can forgive the hyperbole, the mood swings with PMDD are like being pushed on a multi-directional tyre swing by an Austrian powerlifter over a pit of hungry crocodiles. It can be a 360-degree, upside-down, stomach-churning change.

The mood swings can be sudden and powerful, and this volatility makes it difficult to plan events, enjoy certain social occasions, or even just find satisfaction in daily living. Often, those afflicted with PMDD will regularly feel down, overwhelmed, tearful, angry, irritable or even suicidal. Whilst 'in' PMDD – the most minor thing can spiral out of control to become a major incident that makes life feel like it's not worth living –running out of milk at home can go from being a routine domestic non-event to a life-altering existential crisis, leaving a relationship hanging by a thread. Many people unfamiliar with PMDD may read this and think I am exaggerating how severe these symptoms are. I am not exaggerating; I'm just getting started.

The word "dysphoric" means to have a profound or deep dissatisfaction...a word that I could aptly attach to my experiences with Hermes delivery drivers! However, that would be an injustice to both Hermes and the word "dysphoria."
How deep is the dysphoria with PMDD? In the words of Joe Black in the movie "Meet Joe Black," "*multiply it by infinity, and take it to the depth of forever, and you will still have barely a glimpse.*" Yes, the dysphoria can be deep.

The dysphoria permeates every aspect of the sufferer's life in the run up to their period. We all have things in our lives that we feel some dissatisfaction with, but during PMDD, these feelings become overbearing and suffocating. PMDD takes the seeds of hopelessness, anxiety, and catastrophe and keeps inflating them, leaving the person feeling so overwhelmed that life becomes too much to bear, so it's no wonder there is a high incidence of suicide and suicidal thoughts.

Below are some symptoms of PMDD – this isn't a diagnostic criterion, but a snapshot of what someone with PMDD might experience. PMDD symptoms are like a buffet – you can have some or all!

Symptoms of Premenstrual Dysphoric Disorder

Emotional experiences
- mood swings
- feeling upset or tearful
- feeling angry or irritable
- feelings of anxiety
- feeling hopeless
- feelings of tension or being on edge
- difficulty concentrating
- feeling overwhelmed
- lack of energy
- less interest in activities you normally enjoy.
- suicidal feelings

Physical and behavioural experiences
- breast tenderness or swelling
- pain in your muscles and joints.
- headaches
- feeling bloated
- changes in your appetite such as overeating or having specific food cravings.
- sleep problems (sleeping too much or being unable to sleep)
- finding it hard to avoid or resolve conflicts with people around you.
- becoming very upset if you feel that others are rejecting you.

This letter, "if something should happen to me", succinctly describes the cumulative strain PMDD can have on someone's life.

"For my whole adult life, for more than 20 years, I have been struggling to manage with PMDD. The monthly cycle that affects me for about 7 to 10 days out of every 30 I struggle with a debilitating hormonal mood disorder. A third of my life I'm left feeling very much out of control and unable to be myself. I am confronted with emotions that are very often overwhelming. When I'm by myself these feelings are usually feelings of sadness, emptiness, chronic fatigue and hopelessness. Towards my husband, I unfairly expressed agitation and anger. Once the cloud has been lifted, I'm then left with the aftermath of guilt, remorse, shame and self-loathing. Having to then try and find forgiveness from others and for myself. Then comes the dread of what's to come as it all just cycles back around and repeats itself time and time and time again. It's relentless and unforgiving.

I feel by this point I really have tried everything I can to make healthy choices and overcome this the best I can. I've spoken to doctors, therapists and psychiatrists. I have talked with family and friends. Understandably, people don't know what to say or do. They often try to give me words of encouragement and reassurance. To tell me that it can't be that bad. Even the doctors either don't understand, don't know how to treat me or the issue or more commonly, don't believe in the diagnosis itself.

I've spent hours reading books and medical journals to try and better understand the diagnosis. I understand that there's a genetic component to PMDD. I understand that it is not a mental health issue. It is not depression or bipolar disorder. PMDD is a mood disorder due to the brain's abnormal response to the monthly fluctuations of natural chemical hormonal changes. Even though I know this information and I know that it's not my fault, it's medical, physical and genetic, I still feel crazy and out of control. I haven't found any medical professionals with any experience and I often have to educate them about my own diagnosis. There isn't yet the research or treatment available to effectively treat PMDD. Therefore I'm left feeling hopeless.

I try to eat healthy, exercise, socialise and meditate. But the honest truth is these things don't fix the problem and I'm just exhausted from constantly working so hard to keep my head above water.

PMDD is not who I am but it affects who I am every day. It changes my behaviour and how I see the world. It affects every aspect of my life. For years it has sabotaged relationships and friendships. It has put unmanageable stress and strain on my marriage. It has led me to be cruel and unkind. PMDD is also the dominant factor as to why I haven't had children. It has taken my dreams and my life from me. It has robbed me of many opportunities.

A life with PMDD is no life at all. It is not a life that I wish to continue. If I believed that there was a way for these symptoms to be managed, then I could maybe feel hopeful for a positive future. However at this point all I see is a future with more of the same. Months and years of the same symptoms. The only reassurance any doctor has ever given me is that once I reach menopause, many of these symptoms may stop. At 39, it feels like a very long way away and I'm left wishing my life away. By the time I reach menopause in 10 to 15 years, I'm not sure what kind of life I will be left with. I am just not able to be myself. Not able to be the person I truly am. Not able to be the friend and wife I wish to be. I no longer want to be controlled by my erratic brain chemistry.

I need freedom from the overwhelming burden that has me trapped."

– Anon

It is a sobering account of just what it must be like to live with PMDD. It is merciless and recalcitrant. PMDD targets the dreams, expectations, happiness, employment and family relationships of those who have it.

Nothing is sacred, and *nothing* is spared.

Physical symptoms may include a lack of energy, paralysing lethargy, fatigue, and a lack of interest in usual activities. My wife once went for a nap and woke up *still tired* 16 hours later. I kept checking on her to make sure she was still breathing. Trying to get through the day during PMDD for my wife was like wading through thick mud, where it took a monumental effort for the tiniest bit of progress.

Symptoms can start after ovulation (in a typical 28-day cycle, this would be around 2 weeks before the period arrives). So that means your partner might show symptoms for up to two weeks. This is called the "luteal phase" and it is the time that the ovaries, in their benevolence, make a grandiose gesture by "releasing an egg". You see, the ovaries are hoping for something. Each month there is a palpable excitement amongst the sex organs in anticipation of a special event, that, *this might be the month of pregnancy.* The sex organs are hell bent on making their preparations regardless of whether your partner is getting pregnant or not. It is during this phase that premenstrual symptoms can occur.

The Menstrual Cycle

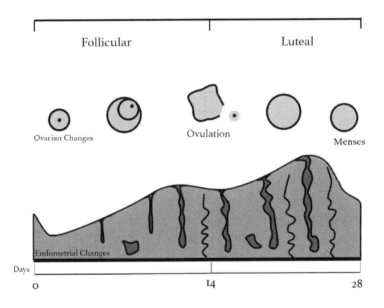

@HopePMDD

Once the egg is **not** fertilised, the excess lining from the uterus is shed in disappointment, and it exits from the vagina. Taa daa, that is what the "period" is. And it is around then that, as if by magic, the symptoms of PMDD should largely dissipate within a few days of the period arriving. This is "menses,"[4] and some PMDDers describe it as a feeling of a "black veil lifting."

Thank heavens for that.

So, why do these symptoms disappear after the period arrives? We don't know, but we know it has something to do with the hormonal fluctuations that occur within the menstrual cycle. We know it's about the chemical messengers in the body, hormones: these are signals the body uses internally to keep its rhythm and its functions in check.

It's not that those with PMDD have a "hormone imbalance" or that they have too much or too little of one particular hormone, it is more about the way the brain interacts with the fluctuations in these hormones. PMDD is about the body having a **sensitivity to hormonal changes**. Progesterone and oestrogen hormones have the largest influence on the symptoms of PMDD. After menopause, the symptoms of PMDD diminish or disappear because the menstrual cycle has disappeared. The menstrual cycle has been decimated, and the body is unable to throw hormones around the way it used to, like confetti at a wedding.
Ultimately, **PMDD is a physiological condition that causes profound psychiatric symptoms.**

PMDD is estimated to affect around 5.5% of the menstruating population, which is about one in 20. That is a massive amount.

---

[4] If the symptoms persist for a whole month, then it may be worth re-evaluating if your partner has other conditions in addition to or instead of PMDD, e.g., Premenstrual Exacerbation (PME). However, everyone is different, and some women still get symptoms for a while after the period arrives. Research is starting to suggest that there might be subtypes of PMDD that express themselves differently. So, if your partner doesn't perfectly fit the traditional symptoms of PMDD, don't worry!

PMDD symptoms can worsen over time or worsen around reproductive events such as pregnancy, birth, miscarriage and perimenopause.[5] Though it's not fully understood why this happens, stress, among other factors, is thought to be implicated.[6]

What causes PMDD?
We don't know.

However, there are (thankfully!) some very clever people trying to work it out. We know that there is a "heritable" or genetic element to PMDD. That means it is likely that it can be passed on through families (30–80% chance), and this heritability has been demonstrated through twin studies.[7] Currently, the main areas that PMDD researchers are looking at (apart from genetic susceptibility) are things that include the structure of the brain or the body's response to specific hormones like progesterone and allopregnanolone. There might also be something going on with what they call the HPA axis. HPA stands for hypothalamus, pituitary, and adrenal glands. If glands were bands, HPA would be the Bee Gees of the body, a tremendous trio.

This is important because not only does the HPA axis regulate the body's stress response, but it also does magic elsewhere in the body, including regulating digestion, the immune system, mood and emotions, sexuality, and energy use. You must stop thinking about parts of the body working separately and see them as fantastically interconnected and interdependent. This is why the spectrum of PMDD symptoms can be so wide ranging.

PMDD stinks, but it's a fascinating medical enigma.

---

[5] https://iapmd.org/about-pmdd
[6] https://faq.iapmd.org/en/articles/4693848-what-can-trigger-pmdd-to-start
[7] https://womensmentalhealth.org/specialty-clinics/pms-and-pmdd/the-etiology-of-pmdd

Two more key areas of research are *serotonin* and *GABA receptors*.[8] I prefer to personalise the neurotransmitter/chemical messenger **serotonin** into a bit more of a personable entity. I call this hormone "Sarah" ..." Sarah Tonin". Sarah helps to moderate mood and irritability, influences memory, and influences people's ability to enjoy things (including libido). Sarah can also influence physical symptoms such as nausea and sickness. Thanks, Sarah, for all that. *It seems that those with PMDD don't seem to respond to serotonin in the same way other people do.* When sex hormone levels are high, serotonin begins to react negatively; it's almost like it misfires. We know that this is one of the reasons SSRI drugs (a type of antidepressant) are particularly useful for PMDD as a first line of treatment. They have been shown to be more effective than a placebo within 24 hours for those with PMDD, which is pretty good![9]

GABA, as mentioned previously, sounds like the name of some sort of space robot, but it's not. There are receptors in the brain that accept a chemical messenger (a neurotransmitter) called GABA. GABA, or 'Gamma-amino Butyric Acid' to give it its full Sunday Best name does all sorts of things. Imagine GABA as a calming hormone; it chills out the nervous system. Anyone who knows anything about PMDD will recognise that there is a distinct *lack* of chill with PMDD. There is about as much chill with PMDD as there is with trench warfare.

Researchers think that it is possible that the GABA receptor isn't working properly in those with PMDD, and so the neurotransmitters don't do their intended purpose of settling the brain and the rest of the nervous system, keeping it in a warzone level of tension. Those with PMDD have something

---

[8] Bixo M, Johansson M, Timby E, Michalski L, Bäckström T. Effects of GABA active steroids in the female brain with a focus on premenstrual dysphoric disorder. J Neuroendocrinol. 2018;30(2):e12553.
[9] Research is the accumulation of lots of people's experience into one set of data. That means that an individual can have a different experience to the conclusions of the research, and it still be valid and useful for others.

going on with nerves and neurotransmitters. That's probably why dental injections aren't as effective for those with PMDD.[10]

Is there more than one subtype of PMDD?

It looks like there may well be. There is a study that analysed the symptom profile of a group of PMDD patients and identified three unique patterns among those patients. Each of the groups seemed to have its own different expression of symptoms. [11]

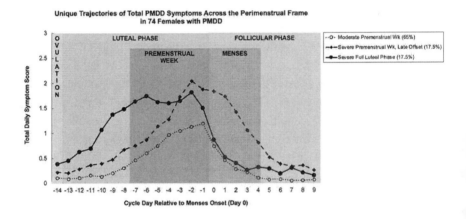

Unique Trajectories of Total PMDD Symptoms Across the Perimenstrual Frame in 74 Females with PMDD

One group reported increased symptoms immediately at ovulation that were sustained and increased towards menses (bleeding), but once the

[10] Mintz M, Badner V, Feldman LK, Mintz P, Saraghi M, Diaz J, Mezhebovsky I, Axelrod I, Gleeson J, Liu C, Smith C, Chow H, Zurakowski D, Segal MM. Lidocaine Ineffectiveness Suggests New Psychopharmacology Drug Target. Psychopharmacol Bull. 2022 Jun 27;52(3):20-30

[11] Tory A. Eisenlohr-Moul *et al.* 2020 *Are there temporal subtypes of premenstrual dysphoric disorder? Using group-based trajectory modelling to identify individual differences in symptom change.* Psychol Med. Reproduced, without alteration under the Creative Commons Licence

period arrived, the **symptoms dropped rapidly** (what the Amazing Dr Tory[12] calls the 'severe full luteal phase').

In the second group, symptoms start at ovulation and gradually ramp up until the period arrives, where they **gradually descend over 3-5 days**. (Inspirational Dr Tory calls this 'severe premenstrual week, late offset')

The last group showed symptoms at a reduced intensity compared to the others and **dropped quite quickly at menses** (Fabulous Dr Tory calls this 'moderate premenstrual week')

---

[12] http://www.toryeisenlohrmoul.com

Making the Diagnosis

PMDD was added to the DSM-5 in 2013. *"What the devil is the 'DSM-5?"* I hear you wail.

The DSM is the *'Diagnostic & Statistical Manual of Mental Disorders'* and it is a massive, fat reference manual that medics, clinicians, and psychiatrists (primarily those in the US) use to arrive at a diagnosis.[13] Up until that point, PMDD had a few different names, including 'late luteal phase dysphoric disorder' but it wasn't fully recognised in a more formal way.

To be diagnosed with PMDD, you must:
- Have five of the 11 specific symptoms they list below.
  - The symptoms occur during the week before menses and improve considerably or disappear once the period arrives.
- Have at least one symptom from the Affective Symptoms list.
- Not be on hormonal birth control or have symptoms attributed to any substance or other disorder.

We know that those with PMDD have abnormal versions of certain genes that process hormones[14] but there is no blood test for PMDD, and the only current way to officially diagnose it is to track those symptoms on a **daily basis** (even on the good days!) for at least two months. If you want some printable trackers, then head here.[15] Or for a digital app, a quick internet search reveals many.

---

[13]   Diagnostic and Statistical Manual of Mental Disorders, 5th ed. Washington, DC: American Psychiatric Association; 2013.

[14]   Dubey N, Hoffman JF, Schuebel K, Yuan Q, Martinez PE, Nieman LK, Rubinow DR, Schmidt PJ, Goldman D. The ESC/E (Z) complex, an effector of response to ovarian steroids, manifests an intrinsic difference in cells from women with premenstrual dysphoric disorder. Mol Psychiatry. 2017;22(8):1172–84.

[15]   https://iapmd.org/symptom-tracker

Affective symptoms:

- lability of affect (e.g. sudden sadness, tearfulness, or sensitivity to rejection)
- irritability, anger, or increased interpersonal conflicts
- depressed mood, hopelessness, or self-deprecating thoughts
- anxiety or tension, feeling "keyed up" or "on edge."

Behavioural/cognitive symptoms:

- decreased interest in usual activities (e.g. work, hobbies, friends, school)
- difficulty concentrating
- lethargy, low energy, easy fatigability
- change in appetite, overeating, food cravings
- Hypersomnia (sleeping too much) or insomnia (being unable to fall or stay asleep)
- feeling overwhelmed or out of control
- physical symptoms (breast tenderness or swelling, headache, joint or muscle pain, bloating, weight gain).

What signs might you notice living with someone with PMDD?

I have previously described the symptoms that someone with PMDD may experience, but now I am going to describe what a partner might notice. From the partner's viewpoint, the symptoms can manifest themselves from a different angle. It is important to note that these symptoms exist only in the luteal phase and subside after the period arrives.

If you are unsure if your loved one has PMDD, then track the cycle and symptom profile of your partner.

If you aren't tracking the cycle, then it's like riding a rollercoaster blindfolded. Tracking is so key. Track and record. Track and learn. Track and prepare. Track, track, trackity track.

The following list might be hard to read for some, but I feel it reflects the reality of what might be observable to a partner of someone with PMDD.

Remember, **these aren't personality traits;** they are manifestations of the symptoms of PMDD that come and go, like a cough during a cold. Your partner during the luteal phase *may* display some of the following:

Heightened irritability: The threshold at which something becomes irritable can be set at zero. Given the right circumstances, your existence, face, and breath can become a source of feverish irritability.

Inflation and exaggeration of negative aspects of life. That thing that was mildly irritating to your partner is now a fundamental, destiny-destroying thing. PMDD takes a sad song and makes it sadder.

Heightened Rejection Sensitivity Dysphoria. There may be a disproportionate response to criticism or rejection. You may feel unable to share negative or positive criticisms with your partner because of the potential for an exaggerated response. When viewed through PMDD glasses, everything appears negative, and your jokes may not land as well as they did before!

Changing views about your relationship: Your partner may express to you that *'you don't deserve me'* but this may flip quickly to *'I don't deserve you'*. It's immensely confusing and cognitively disorienting. If there was a gold medal in mental gymnastics, PMDD would be up on top of the podium, drinking champagne.

Hostile cognitive bias, paranoia, and rumination. Those who have PMDD are more likely to ruminate regardless of where they are in the cycle.[16] Certain negative thought processes may become all-consuming and

---

[16] Kappen et al. Stress and rumination in Premenstrual Syndrome (PMS): Identifying stable and menstrual cycle-related differences in PMS symptom severity. J Affect Disord. 2022 Dec 15;319:580-588.

repetitive, described by my son as the "The Doom Loop". It is difficult to break the destructive narratives and obsessions that can persist. Preoccupations of certain topics that may spring forth like unwanted weeds, e.g. ideations of you being unfaithful, fixations on certain people like co-workers of certain family members/in-laws. Perhaps even simply a preoccupation with certain household habits you have. PMDD normally exaggerates real issues, but it can on occasion, create massively skewed perspectives that reach into the realms of fiction

Intense anger. Rage. Really, really intense - sometimes at everything, but often at **you** in particular. That's a tough blow to be dealt with so frequently. Why are you the lightning rod of rage? I discuss this more later in the book.

Unpredictable Impulsive behaviour. Spontaneous purchases, throwing things out, signing up for things. Not much discussion prior; it just happens.

Propensity to frequently break up the relationship and then reconcile. For some couples, it's every month.

Hypersensitivity to sensory stimuli, e.g. noise, smells, or being touched, especially the sound of you eating. Misophonia (feeling anger, irritation, or stress as a reaction to certain sounds) is commonly reported in those with PMDD; some swear by noise-cancelling headphones or earplugs!

Luteal phase misophonia be like

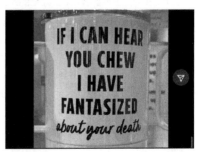

IF I CAN HEAR YOU CHEW I HAVE FANTASIZED *about your death*

Sense of worthlessness, hopelessness There is a fatalistic depression that seems to dispel any future hope of happiness.

Intense fatigue. Sleep can't cure it; it is like every cell in her body has been filled with sand.

Touch feels different. Your touch can be less comforting and can become a trigger. "It's like being touched by sandpaper."

Change in libido. You may find that how sexually appealing you are, has less to do with you and more to do with where your partner is in her cycle.

Baiting involves repeatedly inducing an argument to provoke a response from you. Once you respond by becoming angry- your partner blames you for causing the argument.

Blame and projecting feelings. It is possible that you could experience being blamed for negative events that you aren't really connected to or do not really have any responsibility for. PMDD needs something to attach blame too.

A reduction in empathy or awareness of other people's feelings. Your partner may find it difficult to see past her own viewpoint, experiences, and feelings to consider your viewpoint. It can make you feel like your feelings or wishes shouldn't be expressed or aren't valid.

As you can see from the above list, PMDD causes a considerable and temporary change in a person's disposition. Early on in our relationship I felt I was to blame for (what I now know were) my wife's PMDD symptoms. I decided my approach was to be as perfect as I can; I was going to be absolutely blameless! I worked at perfecting myself for a sustained period of time. Did it make a difference? Maybe a little bit, but not much. I wasn't the cause of the PMDD symptoms, I was a recipient.

The Scale of Change

"My feelings aren't my *decisions,* and my decisions aren't always *my choices.*" Jude Kinghorn.

I spoke with one partner and he shared his PMDD fairytale. "It is like my wife and I are the Queen and King of our castle. We rule there together, and we love each other and rule over our little kingdom. However, for two weeks per month I find I am suddenly marched out of the castle to remain outside its walls whilst being fired upon. I can't get past those walls and I don't understand what is happening inside the castle. Suddenly the doors open and I come inside and it's like the last couple of weeks didn't happen."

The most profound effect of PMDD is the change that is induced in the luteal phase. *A complete shift in gear in terms of mood and outlook.* It can be like dealing with a completely different person whose values, ideals and priorities have shifted dramatically.

We normally think of the mind as separate and independent from the rest of the body, that we electively control our body through our brain, that everything in our life is a direct consequence of every decision we consciously make.

We feel that we are in *absolute control of our body.*

Perhaps it isn't that simple?

Could it be possible that our body can affect our decision making, feelings or even control our brain?

Feelings arrive in our lives like unexpected guests to our body. They weren't invited but they walk through the door regardless. The importance of choice and decision making isn't deciding who arrives, it's about how we treat our guests when they arrive. How do you decide to treat anger when it visits?

If feelings are guests, then having PMDD is like having a travelling zoo break into your house... a tiger coming for tea. The uninvited feelings can be intense, variable, chaotic and they can often make those with PMDD take unusual decisions.

As my wife said confusingly, but wisely, one day, "My feelings aren't my *decisions* and my decisions aren't always *my choices.*"

Think of how your mood can change when you are hungry or "hangry." Our brain and body work together in synergy to achieve the purpose of getting food into us. Your brain says, "I need that delicious taco," and your body says, "Why don't I go and get that for you?" Our body physiology determines a lot more of our behaviour, decision-making, and mood than we think!

PMDD is an extreme case where those normal bodily systems that regulate mood, behaviour, and decision-making malfunction and destructive processes are activated. The body's feedback to the brain is disrupted.

The psychological (and, in some cases, physical) changes that those with PMDD experience vary from person to person. This makes sense, right? Everyone's brain and body are unique and different. Those with PMDD experience it through the lens of their own minds. Symptoms vary from hour to hour, day to day, and month to month. It can leave you as a partner contemplating questions like, "Where does PMDD finish and my partner's character begin?" "Is *my* behaviour the cause of the distress?" "Where are the boundaries of PMDD?" "How do I know what a symptom of PMDD is and what isn't?" "What should I tolerate and what should I not?"

Listening to my wife talk about the thought processes during PMDD, she would explain that sometimes completely irrational behaviour would seem totally rational in that moment. She gave me this example from a few years ago: she was once parking a car in a car park/parking lot and had to reverse into a parking space. She calmly decided that the best way to know how far to go back was just to simply *reverse into the adjacent car,* and once she hit that car, she knew she had reached the perimeter of the parking space.

Now, my wife is very familiar with the generally accepted social norm of society that we do not intentionally drive into other people's cars. However, at the time, it seemed the sensible, logical, and rational thing for her to do, so she did it. [17]

She expressed how beneficial it was as a learning experience for her. She used the event as a reference point to help her recognise how decision-making during PMDD can be altered. Perhaps in that situation, it was easier to recognise the impaired reasoning because there wasn't another person there to influence, complicate, or blame. Cars don't carry the emotional baggage that people and relationships do. There was only my wife, and several inanimate objects.

"My husband would do something minor and I'd get so aggressive and throw things at him...but I was so lonely, too; I was anxious that he didn't love me or find me attractive. I'd scroll through his phone when he was asleep, checking all the apps, his call history, his search history. I even FaceTimed him while he was at work because I was convinced he was having an affair and made him prove to me he wasn't."

Emily

As she talked about it, I imagined myself there, maybe in the passenger seat, trying to convince her that the "reversing into the car" parking method isn't the best. I can imagine it being one of those situations that begins as a minor disagreement and has the potential to become a megadeal.[18]

Have you ever wished there were a crowd of people or hidden cameras to witness the surreal PMDD negotiating predicament you find yourself in? There have been countless situations where, during PMDD, I have found myself feeling helpless, at a loss, trying to explain why a certain course of

---

[17] "No driving offences were committed that day and there was no damage to the other car." Quote Jude Kinghorn 2024

[18] Stylist Magazine - "I want to divorce my husband every month" https://www.stylist.co.uk/health/mental-health/pmdd-premenstrual-dysphoric-disorder-impact-on-relationships/801495

action is undoubtedly misguided. There have been times that I wish my follicular phase wife had been there to back me up!

During PMDD, my wife was prone to throwing things out that we "didn't need." There have been many beloved kids' toys, George Foreman Grills, and clothes that she loved that have been sacrificed on the altar of PMDD. It's just a PMDD "tax," a financial premium that ends up having to be paid.

My wife is an excellent critical thinker, incredibly intelligent, and can juggle mind-bogglingly complex concepts and come to logically sound conclusions. I get carefully thought-out advice from her, and there is no one's opinion I value more than hers. In many ways, this really helped to make a clearer distinction between PMDD-tainted decisions and the carefully considered decisions my wife would normally make.

The gulf between PMDD and non-PMDD was vast and very clearly demarcated as time went on. To me, it was easy to spot when my wife was PMDDing. I could pick up the phone and call her and know within seconds that it had hit; you could hear it in her voice – the tension, the sadness, like the happiness had been sucked from her. In Harry Potter, there are gliding, wraithlike dark creatures called Dementors, which are widely considered to be one of the foulest things to inhabit the world. Dementors feed on human happiness and generate feelings of depression and despair in anyone near them. PMDD, I suppose, is the dementor that visits you both every month for up to a couple of weeks, sucks all the happiness, and then promises to come back in two weeks and do it all again. *The joy of joys.*

"When I am on PMDD time, I hate my partner. I mean, I hate him. I can't stand him. Once I have finished my PMDD time, I will be in love with him again. I don't get it. How can this be normal?"

PMDD warrior, PMDD forum

Her whole demeanour could change, and this could happen instantly. A shift from a chilled-out, happy partner to one who is tense, anxious, depressed, and unflinchingly negative. It wasn't just like someone had emptied her of all happiness; it was like someone had just poured in rancour and bitterness in its place.

It seems like the most negative part of the brain is given a licence to run the whole body. If you were in battle during a war, your brain would be activating differently; your senses would be extremely heightened, you would perceive everything as a threat, and you would be ready to fight at every given moment. PMDD seems to introduce a war-zone mentality into a domestic setting. Perhaps this is why the fatigue with PMDD is so real. To maintain this level of hypersensitivity in a heightened state must be exhausting.

It is no wonder that scientists can identify a brain with PMDD to 74% accuracy simply by doing an MRI scan. Their brains look different.[19]

The problem is, you can't expect someone to just "snap out of it" or heal themselves by "thinking positively." It's like asking someone to fix a broken arm through wishful thinking. My wife struggled to understand why it wasn't possible for her to wake up one morning and simply "take control" and be the person she wanted to be. It was galling to see her disappointment.

---

[19] Differential grey matter structure in women with premenstrual dysphoric disorder: evidence from brain morphometry and data-driven classification. Dubol et al. 2022

Responsibility and Progress

A question is often asked by other partners "How responsible is my partner for her PMDD?" or "How much control does my partner have over PMDD?"

Obviously, your partner is *not* responsible for having PMDD, nor does your partner have control over the occurrence of symptoms. You can't blame someone with a cold for having a cough.

But your partner does have responsibilities in trying to *manage* PMDD. It is reasonable to expect someone to have a degree of ownership over a condition that affects themselves and can exert a damaging effect on loved ones.

What adds to the complexity of answering questions of accountability, is that we are talking about a group of individuals where the inherent nature of their illness *shifts, shapes and reframes.*

British weather is notoriously variable. It sits in the middle of several weather systems that collide together. There is a constant contest for which weather system will prevail. It means each day can be very different from the next. That is why we British are obsessed by the weather and it becomes a focus of so much small talk.

Asking how responsible your partner is for ownership of PMDD is like trying to ask a British person what the weather is going to be like next Tuesday. We'd love to spend some time speculating, but we don't actually know.

Your partner's **capacity, intention** and **accountability** are the key weather systems for ownership of PMDD. They increase and decrease, they expand and contract, they shift and they cycle. The conditions for ownership and progress rely on the intermingling of these following principles:

Capacity

How capable your partner is at a given time.

Accountability

How responsible your partner is at a given time.

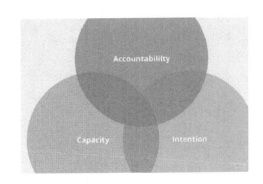

Intention

What your partner really desires/wants

Of course, progress isn't reliant on these factors alone. External factors like; access to healthcare, medications, treatments, a support network etc. are all crucially important.

Capacity

Capacity: How physically or mentally capable your partner is at a given time.

Have you ever seen your partner struggle and frustrated to do simple things? Whether it's brain-fog disrupting a conversation or lethargy that gives such low energy that a trip to the local store may as well be a trip to the moon?

Fatigue, lethargy, depression, anxiety and irritability are symptoms that can reduce someone's *physical capacity*. It might mean that your partner is unable to get out of bed or make phone calls. It might mean a social event is overwhelming. It might mean a performance in a meeting is impaired. It can also be that the reduction in physical capacities can change the mental capacity. If someone can't get out of bed and do the things they want to do, they are more likely to feel depressed, guilty or frustrated. Their PMDD has reduced their capability to function. It is hard to register this change as a by-stander as your partner may look the same. PMDD is a hidden disability.

Mental capacity shifts during points in the luteal phase. One thing that is particularly strange to see as an observer is that during the depths of PMDD, there can be the unleashing of a different 'moral' version of your partner. There could be a skewed version of the values and principles that my wife would normally hold. It didn't reflect who she really was.

I remember once working a long day as a newly qualified professional and volunteering for a youth group one evening per week. One evening after volunteering, I came back late. I was exhausted. It was in the luteal phase and I was run down. My wife had texted me earlier in the day to pick up some milk for the kids breakfast. I came back home and walked through the door. As soon as I walked in the room, it felt charged. I knew the dynamic. I knew the cascade of events that would inevitably unfold.

"Have you remembered the milk?"

I hadn't.

It was as if the world was about to end and the fate of all the citizens of the world was held in the balance by one simple action: remembering the milk.

The reaction was proportional to the sin of destroying the world rather than forgetting the milk. It might sound like I am exaggerating, but I am not.

My wife is an inherently understanding and compassionate person. She is someone who is willing to let the minor things slip when they need to. She is able to contextualise, rationalise and be solution oriented. There was no explanation good enough to rationalise the dysphoria away. In that moment, I had become the conduit for everything wrong about everything.

At that moment my wife was too ill to be able to contextualise the minor discrepancy.

A shift in mental capacity had occurred.

Of course, I could have said at that moment, "Hey Jude, it's not the milk...*it's the hormones*" That would have been a disaster.

"It's just your hormones".

Please, please, please. Never say this.

Using this statement in any argument or discussion has a success rate of zero percent. It is the PMDD equivalent of "calm down".

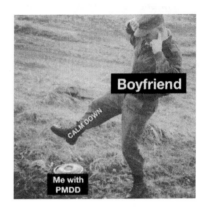

Never in the world was anyone made any calmer by someone telling them to *calm down*.

It is never ever purely hormones alone that reduce capacity. The hormones just seem to ride on the back of pre-existing malcontent. We all have things about our lives that we don't like. I can think of a lot!

Think about your life. What else (apart from PMDD) do you feel ticked off at? Maybe it's a jerk at work, debt, or parenting issues – these are all genuine problems. PMDD takes genuine concerns and keeps inflating them until they become all-encompassing and suffocating. Then, magically, once the period arrives, they deflate and retreat to the psychological back rooms of the mind.

You may notice that trying to discuss PMDD during the luteal phase is an exercise in futility. It doesn't work. Arguments between you and her seem to polarise; the partner is blaming PMDD, while the sufferer looks at her life, and all she sees are valid reasons why she should be unhappy.

She is saying, "It's my life," while the partner is saying, "Look! It's PMDD!"

Logic didn't work and wasn't a useful tool to employ in discussion during the depths of the luteal phase. It feels like you are both in the same world but in a different reality, and the gulf between the two of you is irreconcilable. Whether it is heightened confirmation bias, paranoia or adhering to entirely false narratives, *you can't reason your way out.*

Before becoming angry or upset at the behaviour during PMDD, I tried to put my head in her place and consider the times where I have lost a degree of context, felt overwhelmed, and become acutely angry. So let us do an experiment now. I have wondered if we could replicate the conditions of PMDD in non-sufferers. I am going to try to replicate it through "the sandwich analogy." This analogy is what it might take to bring a person like you or me to the point where we could feel a portion of the awfulness of the luteal phase. However, I totally recognise that this situation wouldn't even *begin* to cover the real feelings of PMDD, but in order to help non-PMDDers understand a little more, it is a useful mental exercise. We all need to step outside our own minds, right?

Let me take you on a mental journey...

The Sandwich Analogy

You take a 24-hour flight to attend a funeral for the death of a close friend; you are already quite sensitive as you are grieving their death. It hits you hard. For some reason, you are bringing the whole family to the funeral, and you end up being the carer to two young children on a very long 24-hour flight. The reason you end up looking after the children alone is that your partner has been upgraded to first class or executive seating on the plane. You did not sleep the night before and cannot sleep on the plane, and the kids don't like the airline food. One child is restless and annoying passengers while the other child is crying incessantly. You hear passengers tutting, and you feel your irritability rising. You imagine your partner sipping champagne in the first-class section of the plane. When you finally land, you wait for an hour for your baggage, only to find the airline has lost all of it. The airport staff can't locate the baggage and are unhelpful and rude. Your partner won't speak to you as she is still angry about you being "cranky on the plane." You are in a different time zone late at night, the airline lost your baggage, you and the kids are hungry and crying, you're sleep deprived and stressed, and you can't find your hotel. You are lost. You are so tired that you feel nauseous. Your phone rings; it's your boss. You are in no state to take a phone call from work, but since it's your boss, you answer it. She fires you. At this point, you are past caring. The phone call ends, and you try to buy a sandwich. Your bank card is declined, but you have enough cash to buy one sandwich to share. The purchase of the sandwich feels like a small victory against a backdrop of awfulness. Outside the shop, your partner bumps into you, and your sandwich falls into the gutter.

You lose it.

You have had enough. You scream at your partner, and to a passersby, it looks like a massive overreaction.

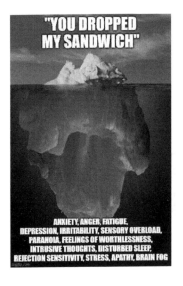

Your partner says, shocked, "Why are you so angry?"

You say, "Because you made me drop my sandwich!"

Is it really "the sandwich"? Not really, but yes.

You are angry. Not just because you dropped a sandwich; you are angry because you are grieving, stressed, tired, hungry, your body clock is off, and you lost your job. You are in an acutely stressful situation. Isn't it completely understandable to feel the way you do?

What is going to be helpful to you in this situation?

Do you feel in the mood to sit down and have a heart-to-heart? No.

Do you want a new damn sandwich? Yes!

Do you want someone to find the hotel for you? Yes!

Will you apologise in a day or two when I have cooled down? Yes, probably.

Will you apologise now? NO!

You don't want to have a heart-to-heart or a root-cause analysis of why you are feeling that way. You are in survival mode. You want to have practical things that are going to relieve you of the stress and make you feel a bit better. You want a sandwich, a hotel room, and to have the funeral over.

If I could borrow your mind for a little longer in our mental gymnastics session, imagine now that you are the person who caused the "sandwich drop." This is most often the position we find ourselves in as partners. We are the ones who are often on the receiving end of all the negative things that happen to our partner. All the anxiety, hatred, and soul-crushing depression that your partner experiences seem to be funnelled towards partners.

You might have done something very simple – a minor mistake – but the reaction is galactically disproportionate.

Obviously, the sandwich was the last straw; the unhappiness had built up over time. But your partner isn't interested in someone pointing out her current state. It is the same reason why a simple inconsequential event can trigger an astonishingly disproportionate unexpected response.

Spilled a glass of water? *"Ha ha, clumsy me."*

Spilled a glass of water? *"My life is a nightmare, I destroy everything I touch, and no one will ever love me."*

Accepting this changed capacity was helpful to me. I stopped adding unhealthy expectations and started to deal with the situation *as it really was*, not what I thought it should be.

I work in the medical field, and whenever we do treatment for a patient, we need their consent. To be able to consent, people need to have the capacity – that is, they must understand the decision and its potential consequences and be free to make the decision. Sometimes people in pain make decisions they wouldn't normally make because the distress they experience clouds their normal decision-making pathways.

There were times when PMDD had made my wife so ill that the capacity to make important decisions or react to a situation was severely reduced.

I presumed, in the early years, if she *"really wanted to,"* she could have improved her condition significantly by self-control alone. *Surely, my wife had some control over her state?* To my shame, I probably felt early on that she just lacked the mental tenacity to deal with normal everyday feelings of tiredness, anger, etc.

I was so wrong.

You need a high mental tenacity to deal with shifts in mental capacity.

Both my wife and I now realise, eight years after her surgery for PMDD (more about that later) that her capacity was reduced to the point that there sometimes was so little or almost nothing she could do to alleviate the symptoms *at that moment.*

My wife would spend two weeks trying to condition herself mentally prior to the PMDD onset to think, "I just won't get angry" or "Mind over matter." Then, when the luteal phase hit, she would feel desperately disappointed and guilty when her pre-luteal conditioning didn't work. Her efforts were in vain, engulfed in the dark clouds of PMDD.

As a rule, big decisions are best avoided in the luteal phase ... for everyone involved. There may be decisions that you consider eccentric or unwise, it doesn't necessarily mean that your partner lacks the capacity to make the decision or is wrong.

Ask yourself if your partner was **not** in the luteal phase:

- Would your partner normally make this decision?
- Are the decisions they make consistent with the values and principles they operate on?
- Are the decisions your partner makes harmful to them and/or those around them?
- Can your partner balance information out adequately enough to come to a reasonable decision?

Most decisions your partner makes, you can't do much about, even if you disagree. However, if the decision is harmful to your partner or to those around them or particularly self-destructive like quitting a job or sending an incendiary message then trying to persuade your partner to hold-off may be a good call. At the very extreme end you may have to call in professional help if the decision is particularly destructive or harmful. e.g. self-harm or suicide attempts.

Once both partners and sufferers accept the extent to which PMDD can temporarily change a person's capacity, work can begin on finding *what can be done and when.*

Accountability

Accountability: How responsible your partner is at a given time for their actions and how able they are to give an account for them.

In this book, I am emphasising *your* role and maximising *your* influence on PMDD. However, in emphasising your influence on PMDD, I do not want to make you think that those who have PMDD are not still ultimately responsible for trying to take as much ownership of the condition as they can.

I have emphasised how little control my wife had over PMDD. But control, capacity and accountability ebb and flow depending on where someone is in the cycle. Two days before the period arrives, capacity is *different* to what it is seven days later.
That is why you can't measure accountability one day to the next; it needs to be measured *over time*. We don't measure climate change based on a single day; we measure it by the sustained patterns in weather systems. Accountability with PMDD is about *intention and trajectory-* which direction does your partner *want* to go and how they are getting there.

When all is said and done, the person who *has* PMDD is the person that *owns* PMDD and that means that you should expect your partner, if she is diagnosed, to be **actively engaging** with the diagnosis and treatment.

47

What other signs of engagement might you see? What is reasonable to expect from someone who has PMDD? The following list is a realistic wish list of what can be reasonably expected from someone who is actively engaged.

- Acknowledge the condition.
- Track the cycle and keep you updated.
- Attend medical appointments
- Seek and trial different treatment options
- Discuss feelings reflectively in the follicular phase
- Show introspection around PMDD behaviours
- Acknowledge impacts of PMDD on those around them and try to reduce harm to others.
- Actively contribute to the relationship when occasion allows.

Your partner does not have control over if she has PMDD symptoms. Yes, positive interventions may be able to reduce the severity of symptoms, but the items listed previously are not symptoms of PMDD, they are positive behaviours that can exist independently of symptoms.

Over the years despite symptoms worsening for my wife, her engagement, accountability for the condition and awareness of how PMDD was influencing her increased massively.

A healthy relationship must have compassionate accountability for the effect of PMDD.

Your partner's accountability is dependent on their capacity. Capacity is the ability

"I had to explain to my partner today that my PMDD basically makes me similar to a drunk person... when I'm in the middle of a rage or depressive episode, I cannot be rationalized with, and I need him to see it that way. You wouldn't try to have a serious conversation with a drunk person...even if they say they can and I'm pretty dang similar. They can't snap their fingers and be sober, and I can't snap mine and instantly become calm and rational. I hate pmdd but this analogy really helped him"

PMDD warrior, PMDD forum

to make informed decisions and be able to carry them through.

If your partner is suicidal, then there has been a sudden plummet in your partner's capacity and you may need to step in to help keep her safe.

Drops in capacity might mean your partner has difficulty recognising PMDD is causing an interpersonal conflict.

Reductions in your partners capacity are opportunities to increase your accountability to your partner. We will look later in the book at ways to help her help herself.

Intention

Without acknowledgement of PMDD by your partner and the intention to improve, it is going to be a difficult journey. In fact, the plain truth is- things probably won't get much better. However again, without the other principles of capacity and accountability, intention is just a nice thought. Capacity & accountability are where the action comes in.

I have encountered many partners who are in a never ending 'Doom Loop' where the same thing is happening over and over. Their PMDD partner does not show any intention to change or seek help, and the partner just deals with the fall-out every month. The person with PMDD fails to recognise the impact or intentionally ignores the problems they are experiencing. Even worse in some cases, where the self-awareness of PMDD is so low, the partner is blamed for the PMDD problems.

The denial of PMDD, whether it is unintentional or subconscious, produces the same results: bitterness and baggage between the two parties. This bitterness becomes more and more entrenched with time and once other friends or family get involved, it is difficult to climb out of the hole that has been dug.

It is the worst of the worst situations. This truly is a vicious cycle.

The biggest influence on the success of a PMDD relationship, in my opinion, **is when the person with PMDD is actively engaged with the diagnosis.** They want to get better as they know they aren't well.

If your partner is *not* engaged with the diagnosis or is in a state of denial, then head to Section 3 where we discuss "Denying the Cycle."

Where there is no intention, there will be no progress. If there is no progress, there is the risk of dangerous situations. Untreated severe PMDD can be extremely damaging to the person with PMDD *and* to their partner.

If PMDD can be severe enough for someone to harm themselves by suicide, then PMDD can be severe enough for someone to become abusive. Am I saying that everyone who has PMDD is abusive? No.
Am I saying that PMDD can create conditions where abuse can exist or even flourish? Yes.
PMDD isn't an excuse for abuse, but it could be part of the reason.

Journalist and author Shalene Gupta wrote in her book *The Cycle: Confronting the Pain of Periods and PMDD*[20]

"During interviews, several people I talked to mentioned struggling with rage. A few said they were abusive towards partners but didn't describe what kind of abuse. I sympathized- rage is difficult to talk about, even more than suicide. It's far easier to admit to being hurt than to hurting someone. People would tell me all about their suicide attempts but then gloss over rage, a sentiment I understood. Society seems to find a woman's death more acceptable than her rage."

PMDD is not a blank cheque to allow persistent damaging behaviours.
If the same thing is happening over and over and your partner is not willing to change or recognise the impact or harm on others, then the relationship will not be sustainable and won't be safe. Improvements come usually with medical treatment. That is why the secondary goal after your partner is actively engaged with the diagnosis is **finding a competent medical professional** who understands PMDD so that appropriate treatment can be offered.

---

[20] Shalene Gupta *The Cycle: Confronting the Pain of Periods, and PMDD. Flatiron Books. Advance reader's edition 2023*

"Insanity is doing the
same thing over and
over and expecting
different results."

Albert Einstein

Mookie's Model of PMDD Progress

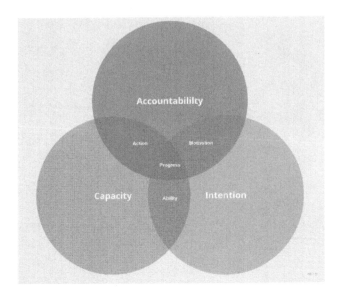

This Venn model really shows the interplay between these three key principles- *Accountability, Intention* and *Capacity*. I named the model after my cat Mookie, who has absolutely no capability or capacity and only seems to have questionable intentions. I swear she is plotting to harm my oldest daughter.

These are *'principles'* we are talking about here. Principles are universal truths that are applied to multiple different scenarios- they aren't very situation specific. Just in the same way the legal system takes the principles of justice and fairness and applies them to individual circumstances, you are going to have to take these principles described in the model and apply them to your unique PMDD relationship.

These are the key ingredients for progress that we have already discussed: capacity, intention and accountability. Let's play around with the ingredients.

You see at the very centre of the diagram is *progress*. *Progress* arrives when those principles work together. Each one is crucial. If there is no **intention** to change or to work with PMDD, then things just won't work as there is no motivation for change- *what does your partner want and where do they want to go?*

If your partner is fundamentally not aligned to be in a relationship with you and this is a core belief, then a relationship is not going to work. Similarly, if your partner has no desire or intention to seek treatment, then there won't be any progress. Intention is the fuel for change. Intention and desire are normally born from education and awareness of the condition and how it affects themselves and others around them.

By combining **intention** along with **accountability,** you get a road map of *what* needs to change. Accountability with PMDD must be empathetic, many things with PMDD are outside the sufferer's control.

Accountability is aspirational in nature, it gives us a wish-list; it gives us something to strive for. Your partner may hold herself accountable by making her own wish-list or goals. Perhaps it could be improvements planning for the luteal phase or seeking out medical treatments; it could be engaging together in couple's therapy. It might also be about reflecting when things haven't gone well and trying to provide an account of her experience.

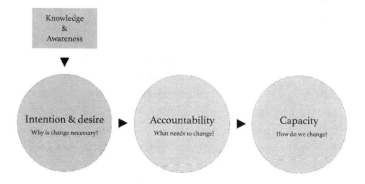

I am sure you both will have a list of what you would like to see improve. What are the things your partner can do to help the relationship become sustainable? Could it be that the impact of verbal abuse is chronically damaging the relationship? Accountability is understanding the gulf between the current situation and the end point.

Knowing that something needs to change provides the *motivation* to progress. But, if there is no **capacity** to turn the aspiration to action, then there won't be progress. Again, you need all three ingredients.

For example, your partner wants to get better (intention) and your partner recognises her role in owning the condition (accountability) and so she is motivated to seek medical care. However, her symptoms are so profound during the luteal phase that she cannot tolerate appointments, phone calls or self-advocating the medical system (capacity). Your partner is willing but not able. In this case it is: *Intention + accountability - capacity= little progress*

Alternatively, your partner may have **capacity** and **accountability**, she may recognise the impact and be able to take *action-* but without **intention** there is no *motivation* and sense of responsibility to make that progress. That would be classed as wilful neglect.

For example, your partner is able, but not willing. Perhaps the relationship is at rock bottom, symptoms have subsided during the follicular phase, but things are so strained your partner does not want to invest in the relationship.

Progress is rarely linear. Most of what has been discussed so far in this chapter is firmly within the ownership of those who have PMDD. These are mostly principles that have to be harnessed internally by the person with PMDD, but you can help with each aspect. For example: You can pick up the slack when your partner is less capable. You can help with intentions by making your relationship worth it. You can help to communicate the impact of PMDD on you and so accountability increases along with motivation for change.

For a moment look at Mookie's model through your own eyes. You have your own version of this model with your own intentions, capability and accountability. Your diagram and her diagram bisect and interconnect! They work together for progress in synergy. Consider just how these principles work for you. Do you have your own issues that affect your capacity? Are you holding yourself accountable for your own actions? Are you committed to the relationship (intention)? As always with relationships, it is a joint effort, both parties doing the best they can.

The Partner Experience

I once had a really bad cough, one of those coughs where it felt like someone stuffed your trachea with sandpaper and punched you in the diaphragm. It was really bad, and I felt sorry for myself. I started coughing, and after catching my breath, I turned to my wife and exclaimed, "This cough is horrendous." At that moment, I looked towards my wife, who returned my look with a death stare. Why?
She was in the middle of a painful labour with our second child.

The suffering that we were experiencing was markedly different at that time. I had a bad cough, and she was pushing a baby out of her body. One of these things is not like the other; one of these things is more painful than the other! Twelve years later, I still occasionally exclaim, "This cough is horrendous." We still laugh about it, but I think I find it slightly funnier than she does.

This is how it feels to be a partner in some ways, you don't want to talk about it because your partner has it a lot worse. You feel sometimes that your suffering, though real, is lessened because someone next to you is suffering more. You might feel that your voice is lost and that you have no right to express those feelings.

You might also keep your own expressions of pain hidden or out of the way. You might feel restrained to secrecy because you do not want to add to the guilt they already have about the way PMDD affects you.

I found that my wife didn't want to hear about my own difficulties. Each phase had its own reasons. Jude will talk now eight years post-surgery about how during the luteal phase she didn't care what I thought or felt. My feelings or difficulties were irrelevant, because I was to blame and I was responsible for her rage and her unhappiness. Why should I complain about my own difficulties when I had manufactured them myself?

During the sobering follicular phase, the reasons were different. It wasn't that she didn't care, in fact, it was the opposite: she cared so much for me that she couldn't bear to hear the suffering that her PMDD was causing. The shame and guilt were weighty.

The true acknowledgement of the impact it was having on those around her was a burden too great to have on top of what she was feeling. Perhaps you don't want to express your true feelings because you are worried about the consequences. What will she say? What will she do?

Everyone has the right to freedom of expression, to speak their truth, and to say how they feel. That's important, right? You deserve to be understood. If you can't talk it over with your partner, you can talk it over with a friend, right? That's not simple either.

Consider how your partner would feel if you started talking frankly to someone else about how things are at home without her consent. PMDD is often so hidden; masking can make it seem to others like nothing is going on.

How comfortable your partner is about talking with others will depend on what stage of engagement your partner has with the diagnosis. For many, especially early on, the PMDD experience is something kept intensely private and can feel deeply personal... like sharing a dark secret. Those feelings are often linked to guilt and shame felt by those with PMDD. For the accompanying partner, it can feel like a breach of confidence to talk about it with friends, family, or even professionals.

I spoke with one partner who shared the same social group as his wife with PMDD. On one trip with some male friends, he confided about some of the difficulties of living with someone with PMDD, sharing with them what would regularly happen at home. Those friends told their wives and soon the whole social group was aware of the PMDD situation. Sometime later, the couple realised that they were no longer being invited to the same social functions that they had been previously. After the partner inquired, it was revealed that the exclusion socially was because they did not feel comfortable with the way he was being treated by his wife.

It is just this type of misunderstanding and discrimination that people worry about. Conversely, both my wife and I have had more positive personal experiences speaking about PMDD than negative ones.

Being the partner of someone with PMDD means you don't own the condition. You can't take the medicine for it, you can't see the doctor for it, and you can't totally understand what it's like to have it.

You don't own it.

It is perplexing that someone else's health condition can have such an impact. Your ability to improve the situation depends to a large extent on the willingness of your partner. It can be frustrating to feel like you can't truly own the problem or take control of it.

At a support group I once attended, the mother of someone with PMDD said something that has stayed with me.
"You partners have a choice." she said, "You can stay, or you can leave your partner. But me? I am her mother, and I can never leave. I can never give up on her. She is my daughter."

Love, it seems, takes us to the extremes of life.

For a moment in this section, just temporarily, I would like to continue to focus on what it is like to be a partner. As hard as it is, we are going to exclude the suffering of those who have PMDD and focus on our own. This doesn't diminish their suffering; it's just defining our own. Every voice that suffers in some way needs to speak, and the route to harmony is understanding where each person's vantage point lies.

While writing about how I felt is cathartic, my reason for writing the following is less about me and more about *you*. From my experience talking with other partners, the commonality of experience is remarkably consistent.

The Impact of PMDD

So how would it begin? Initially, I would feel surprised. It doesn't matter how many years I lived with PMDD; every time the luteal phase started, it caught me off guard.

Every single time.

We would normally be going about our daily business, pottering around in the kitchen, when *something* would happen. It would usually be a small thing, a minor incident, and the **reaction would be disproportionate**. Very disproportionate. There would be an unusual amount of anger for something so mundane and uneventful. For example, my jokes suddenly stopped being funny and became offensive.

Her demeanour and facial expressions would change, unprompted by any event or situation. If people have an aura, then hers had turned black. I don't think it's an exaggeration to say that it felt like she could sometimes be a different person altogether. I would notice that she would become critical of everything I did, picking up on the most minor things, and I would feel like she was trying to entice me into an argument; she wanted to fight! There was a slow burn, an undertone of escalating anger and frustration; my well-intentioned actions would only fuel the negative narrative.
If I tried to help, it didn't.
If I didn't try and help, then I was abandoning her.
I would keep my cool, try to de-escalate, but regardless, often it did not appease the festering malcontent.

The vindictive deconstruction of my character was routine. I am already acutely aware of my failings and weaknesses, so having them as the hot topic of the week was draining. If I gave in and finally offered even the smallest retort, then it would be an explosive and awful experience for everyone. It led me to feel that I was walking on eggshells, uncertain if an innocuous action would spark a fallout. I would second guess everything I said, wondering how it might be interpreted, uncertain about my decisions.

I would become emotionally fatigued, sometimes numb, sometimes angry, but with nowhere for the anger to go. Not every month was like this, but it wasn't infrequent.

At one point, my wife would be happy, content, and having fun, and the next day she would be in a spiralling depressional crisis. PMDD is so cruel, and the grief is so real. When people die, they disappear, and you miss them. They are gone.

When your loved one is PMDDing, they are still with you, but you still grieve the absence of your normally loving partner and long for their return. But while you grieve their absence, you become a receptacle for the anger and irritability of the condition. It's like putting salt in a fresh wound – a new level of heartache. Grief is the price you pay for loving someone. Sometimes it's after a break-up, sometimes it's when they die.

The grief that happens with PMDD happens whilst you are together.

PMDD takes the very person you love the most and turns them against you.

"Grief, I have learned, is really just love. It's all the love you want to give but cannot. All that unspent love gathers up in the corners of your eyes, the lump in your throat, and that hollow part of your chest. Grief is just love with no place to go."
Jamie Anderson

I hung on to what I knew. I knew who my wife really was. I knew PMDD was why she reacted in a certain way. I knew it didn't represent who she really was.

My wife is a kind, loving woman with whom I want to spend my life. Outside PMDD she would never ever behave this way. This wasn't Stockholm Syndrome where people sympathise with their abuser. This wasn't some sort of psychological trick or coping mechanism. It was a factual description of our scenario. I was living with two versions of the same person, one with PMDD and one without, and they were *completely different.*

At the beginning of our relationship, I knew that something was different, but I didn't know what. I also wondered if every relationship was like this, and everyone else was having the same experience in secret.

It was an intense and immensely confusing time in the early years of the relationship. I was on a psychological rollercoaster with my wife; we were riding this thing together, and we didn't know it. We were having some good times (the ups) and very considerable 'drops.' We didn't realise there was a pattern.

We were arguing over bizarre things that didn't really matter. As time went on, like many partners, I developed a thick skin and a lot of patience, but the gains came at significant costs. In the early years of PMDD, I lost a lot of confidence and I felt, at times, worthless; it permeated my job, other relationships, and my outlook on life. It felt like my spark and my zest for life had gone, and I was the cause of my wife's unhappiness. I had always felt like an honest, decent, well-meaning person who wanted more than anything for her to be happy. It was hard to reconcile that, despite my endeavours to be the most loving, perfect husband I could be, I seemed to be the source of everything wrong about her life.[21]

As my behaviour was assigned as the source of her unhappiness, I started to consider if I were a really awful person with a lack of self-awareness. During the acute stages of PMDD, my wife would say some hurtful things, words that hurt more and penetrate deeper because they came from someone I love so deeply. The verbal abuse was intensely personal and sustained, and no topic was too sacred for PMDD to desecrate. Even now, years later, it is upsetting to think of these moments.

I consider myself to be naturally robust with a high degree of tenacity. I have been lucky to have always had good health, both mentally and physically. These aren't things I credit to myself; more, I have always been resilient and consider it a part of my physiology. I am grateful for this because I feel that if I or my wife had any additional mental health

---

[21] For more information on the impact of PMDD in partners see Appendix B which contains the results of a survey of almost 100 partners.

problems, addictions, or substance abuse difficulties (this list is not exhaustive!) the strain would have been too much for me. PMDD will exploit any vulnerability within you or in the relationship. After all, PMDD exaggerates and inflates any negative thing it can.

I would wishfully look at other couples and families with envy – imagine having a partner who is able to show their love consistently or who has the energy to go out and about with the children? My wife would be in bed for much of the weekend or evenings during PMDD, in a stupor of sleep or depression. Raising four children takes work. It was galling to read the stereotyping in the media about "men" who failed to do housework or help with childcare duties. I was working full-time, cleaning, cooking, entertaining, doing homework, shopping, and dealing with the difficulties of PMDD in the process. I have always been a hands-on dad and do not subscribe to the Victorian-distant-fatherhood model, but this was extreme parenting under war zone-like conditions. It was like parenting under machine-gun fire.

During PMDD, I would be very lonely. I ached for the affection my wife would normally show, and I longed to have her back. I wished someone knew or understood what we were going through, and I wished I could talk to someone. I felt angry at times that this was happening to her and me. I felt helpless, especially in the early stages when she was not undergoing any treatment and lacked insight during the luteal phase into the behavioural symptoms. I talked to no-one. My children could be the antidote. We would flee to the local playground or run in the woods. The unconditional love of a child reaches deep and lifts so high. They have no idea of the strength they have been to me.

I was at one point quite an ambitious person; my career had started out very well, and my trajectory was one of rising to the top of my profession. I wanted to be someone who would leave his mark on the world, but I realised that my energies would have to be primarily directed to where they were needed most, which was caring for my wife and children. I found a new purpose in being a caregiver. I have no regrets about taking this direction, but I do not judge anyone who comes to a different position; we each know our capacities and what we can deal with.

Getting through PMDD deepened the understanding and communication Jude and I had together. Coming out of the other end of PMDD, I feel that we are stronger and more understanding of each other than we would have otherwise been. I feel like the most worthwhile things in life have a cost, either in time, money, mental exertion, or emotion. A PMDD relationship came at a high cost, but it made it infinitely more valuable to me.

I was and am happy to pay the price for what I have today.

I totally understand, though, for some partners, the relationship has such high a price tag that it becomes unaffordable. Sometimes a relationship can't work no matter how much you invest.

Diagnosis and Treatments

If you are reading this, then you must have gotten to the point where one of you in the relationship has recognised signs or symptoms of PMDD. Perhaps your partner has been formally diagnosed? This is a big win! For most of those who have PMDD, it can take years and years until a diagnosis of PMDD is made.

Some research in the United Kingdom showed that PMDD patients took an average of 12 years for an accurate diagnosis and saw 11 healthcare providers in the process.[22] It's even more of a big win if your partner, who suffers from PMDD, understands it and is willing to engage in efforts to improve the condition. **The ultimate PMDD jackpot (is there such a thing as a PMDD jackpot?) is having a good doctor who understands PMDD.**

By far the most effective thing someone who has PMDD can do is to get *effective treatment from a competent specialist medical professional that understands PMDD.*

Everything else is an appendage to this. As hard as that individual may be to find, the key words remain **effective, competent, and understanding.**

I spent four years with my wife before we recognised that the pattern of behaviour followed the menstrual cycle. How this simple fact evaded us feels utterly humiliating; looking back, it seems so obvious. However, being oblivious to the obvious does seem to be a pattern of behaviour for both of us, particularly me. This is evidenced by the fact that we owned a family car for almost two years before realising it had a sixth gear. We had been

---

[22] Divine, M., Ozturk, S., Kania, A., Buchert, B.,, Wagner-Schuman, M., Miller,A.,. & Eisenlohr-Moul, T. (2019). Lifetime Prevalence of Self-Injurious Thoughts and Behaviours in a Sample of 591 Patients Reporting a Prospective Clinical Diagnosis of Premenstrual Dysphoric Disorder BMC Psychiatry 2022

travelling the breadth of the country in 5th, not realising there was an 'extra' gear.

It is a testament to how much periods, the menstrual cycle, and women's health are largely overlooked in society that both myself and my wife had never heard of PMDD or knew little about how PMS or mood changes are related to the menstrual cycle. We both had a mild awareness that it was possible that mood changes could occur prior to menstruation, but that was it. Pretty basic.

Once we realised what PMDD was, it was like someone switched on a massive light in my life, often described as 'the light bulb moment' by those who experience it. Like Neo in the movie The Matrix. I could see everything exactly for what it was, and I could understand what was happening. Just like Neo, once we understood the rules of what was happening, we could start to take some control. It didn't give us immunity from harm, but knowing about PMDD meant there were a few bullets we could dodge. There was a clearly defined pattern staring us in the face. Literally within a day of the period arriving, I had my loving, kind wife back. (though tainted with the psychological trauma of what she experienced in luteal phase).

My wife and I both accepted that the symptoms she was experiencing were so intense that further medical advice and investigation were needed. My wife had been reluctant to see a professional initially, but after two years of monitoring cycles, things had gotten worse. She was visiting the family doctor for another reason, so I encouraged her to mention her experiences. She was fearful of being dismissed, ignored, belittled, or humiliated. Her creeping self-doubt told her that she would be labelled a fraud, a hypochondriac, or ignored.

I found it bizarre that she felt like this, given how significant her symptoms were, but perhaps this uncertainty in speaking up reflects how men and women are sometimes treated or listened to differently. Perhaps this is why it has taken so long for the medical profession to take this condition seriously. Medicine, which was traditionally a male-dominated, "doctor knows best" profession, is now becoming more "patient-centred" and gender-balanced. This means that women are more likely to be listened to and heard, hopefully. However, there is still a lack of knowledge about premenstrual disorders in the medical profession. It is a shame that for a person to gain a diagnosis of PMDD, it can take as long as it does.

That's where you come in. Research shows that if a patient receiving medical care has an 'advocate,' then the standard of care provided improves (*with your partner's consent,* this can be one of your roles). You can be her supporter, her advocate, and her team. You can be the person to encourage and reinforce the constructive behaviours in seeking medical care that otherwise her self-doubt might strangle. Of course, care must be taken that you remain in the passenger seat, helping to navigate rather than trying to dominate or take the wheel. Your partner must be the one executing the decisions; after all, it is her body and her health condition.

I also appreciate the stress and emotional strain that you already experience. In the survey I performed, 73%[23] of partners noted that their partner's PMDD had a *considerable* or *extreme* effect on their own mental health. Finding the resolve to help another when you are suffering in your own way is difficult but noble.

It is also, bizarrely, a way that you can strengthen the relationship longer term. By making PMDD the common enemy and working together, you may deepen your levels of communication and trust. Crucially, it is a way you can improve the life of the one you love while simultaneously improving your own.

My wife recounted that at her doctor's appointment, she had discussed the primary reason for her visit, and just before she left, almost as she was walking out the door, she mentioned (very briefly and hesitantly) some of the symptoms she was experiencing before her period arrived. The doctor (who, as it turns out, had a special interest in menstrual disorders) leapt onto the subject and asked her more questions, listened to the answers, gave options, and arranged a follow-up.

THANK THE LORD ABOVE FOR THAT DOCTOR. If I were the shrine-building type, there would be a carefully sculpted granite structure of that

---

[23] Full survey results included at the end of the book.

doctor in my back garden, to which I would make a daily pilgrimage to leave flowers and poems and scented candles.

I was so relieved. My wife felt great. Shrine or not, I still have an abiding love for that doctor, who effectively changed the course of our lives. This is the difference a professional can make. They can change the course of someone's life. A medical professional who really listens to their patients is deserving of the place in society in which they are held. We were incredibly lucky and recognise that this is not what a lot of people experience. For many women, the rights of passage seem to be a twisted journey of being misdiagnosed, ignored, and medically gaslighted.

PMDD is poorly recognised worldwide, and only recently have treatment options been developed. Thankfully, there is *some* research into the outcomes of different treatment options. Like many other conditions, the treatment of PMDD depends on its severity.

The Royal College of Obstetricians and Gynaecologists in the UK has published guidance on the management of Premenstrual Syndrome, which, although not specific to PMDD, offers at least a pathway or reference. Though meant as guidance to doctors, the guidance is helpful to partners and patients for an overview of the diagnosis and treatment options for PMDD.[24] Additionally, the American College of Obstetricians and Gynecologists[25] in 2023 published guidelines.[26]

Additionally, I can recommend you visit the website of the IAPMD[27] (International Association for Premenstrual Disorders), who are the overlords of information and goodness on PMDD and PME on the world wide web. Conventional wisdom might dictate that IAPMD is run by normal humans, but it isn't, IAPMD is run by angels. They are fabulous, and if I were to construct a second shrine in my backyard, it might be to

---

[24] Premenstrual Syndrome, Management (Green-top Guideline No. 48) | RCOG https://www.rcog.org.uk/guidance/browse-all-guidance/green-top-guidelines/premenstrual-syndrome-management-green-top-guideline-no-48/

[25] ACOG Press release https://www.acog.org/news/news-articles/2023/11/acog-releases-new-guidelines-on-management-of-premenstrual-disorders

[26] ACOG Clinical Guidelines: https://www.acog.org/clinical/clinical-guidance/clinical-practice-guideline/articles/2023/12/management-of-premenstrual-disorders

[27] International Association for Premenstrual Disorders https://iapmd.org/

them and their wonderful work. Co-founder of IAPMD, Sandi MacDonald is the epitome of all that is good in the world and her relentless perseverance in serving those who have PMDD is the stuff of legends.

I would really recommend looking at the resources available on their website for contemporary, evidence-based guidance. I will give a very brief overview of just some of the mainstream treatments that are available. What I write isn't medical advice but more of a signal to you and your partner to realise that there are treatments available and that some women have had success with one or a few of them. They can be life-changing for those who respond well to the treatments. The unfortunate truth is, though, that many treatments just aren't specific or effective enough for PMDD, and treatment needs to be better. However, the message of modern medicine is there is hope!

How is PMDD diagnosed and treated?

There are no blood tests, scans, or chemical markers that are used to make a diagnosis of PMDD. As pointed out previously in the book, the diagnosis of PMDD is made based on a record of the symptoms, and the person is asked to keep a diary and to record their symptoms over two cycles. This diary shouldn't be performed afterwards, as looking back retrospectively is less reliable than recalling symptoms as you go.

Given the rare understanding of PMDD and the relative inexperience most family doctors have in treating it, many will refer the person suffering from PMDD to a specialist doctor or gynaecologist after trying first-line interventions, e.g. exercise, diet, cognitive behavioural therapy (CBT), SSRIs (antidepressants), etc. The specialist will normally take things further and explore the more advanced options for managing PMDD. Sometimes, if the symptom diary is inconclusive and there is a lack of certainty surrounding a diagnosis of PMDD, the gynaecologist may prescribe a three-month course of a medication called "GnRH analogues." This is a medication that suppresses the production of the hormones used in the menstrual cycle, a so-called *"chemical menopause."* Remember, **PMDD is a hypersensitivity to changes in these hormones**, and by flattening them off or suppressing the levels of certain hormones, someone with PMDD should find that the PMDD symptoms reduce. It's not permanent, and if the person stops taking the medication, then the cycle returns to normal in time.

The best place to look for a contemporary synopsis of current treatment options isn't my ramblings here on treatment options; it is from the IAPMD, those heaven-sent angelic earth-walkers who have been at it again in producing a comprehensive and carefully considered guide to treatment options: https://iapmd.org/treatment-options

Nonetheless, here is a little taste of some treatments:

First line treatments

Among the first lines of treatment will likely be diet, exercise, and cognitive behavioural therapy (CBT). Your family doctor/GP may expect your partner to work on these interventions before any pharmacological (drug) treatment is considered. Many people do have success with them. Keeping a **healthy diet and exercising** regularly have been shown in research to improve people's moods and overall well-being. Not just people with PMDD, but everyone, including you.

This may be enough for your partner; great! But for many, it is not. In my own experience, despite monumental efforts being made to control the diet and get more exercise, my wife's PMDD was so severe that exercise and diet offered little discernible change to her wellbeing during the premenstrual phase.

Cognitive Behavioural Therapy (CBT) is a talking therapy that aims to help people manage their problems by changing the way they approach or think about things.

Everybody should use CBT; it seems to help everyone in some way. CBT is the multi-tool/Leatherman of psychological interventions, a tool that can be used to help a wide range of problems. It's normally accessible through your doctor, or there are private providers who can be found through a quick Google search. It may be worthwhile to be selective (if you are afforded that choice) and see a therapist who understands the biological reality of PMDD and does not simply see it as a 'psychological problem' that can be fixed completely by changing learned behaviours. PMDD is more complex than that. It is my personal view that there is an overreliance on therapy as a treatment for PMDD. Though therapy can make a great difference for many sufferers, fundamentally, you can't simply think or "choose" your way out of PMDD. Like many of the interventions for PMDD, therapy is a crucial ingredient in the recipe for PMDD treatment, but it is not the whole cake. CBT can be a great way to help contextualise, process, and manage the symptoms in a better way. Who is ever not going to benefit from CBT?

Ironically, these first-line treatments – diet, exercise, and CBT – are very useful not just for PMDD sufferers but for their partners as well. Trying to cope with the emotional, mental, and physical strain of PMDD will place great demands on your health. In my survey, almost sixty percent of partners reported a negative impact on their physical health from their partner's PMDD. Recognise that you may need support or improvements in your diet, exercise, or perhaps therapy or medication. It is my opinion that the strain of living alongside someone who has PMDD means that every partner should be actively undergoing therapy or formal support to help them cope with caring for or living with someone who has PMDD.

I should put a massive proviso in this text when talking about treatment options for PMDD: **EVERYONE IS DIFFERENT**. Just because something works for someone doesn't mean it will work for you, and vice versa. Consider that each person's unique physiology means their experience of an intervention may be different from others'. As pointed out previously there is the possibility that there may be different subgroups of PMDD. This means, for example, that some of those with PMDD symptoms will have symptoms that last a few days into their period, whereas others' symptoms stop immediately once the period arrives.

Pharmacological Interventions
SSRIs
SSRIs are one of the first lines of treatment for PMDD. They are called selective serotonin reuptake inhibitors. You might remember Sarah from earlier on in the book. Sarah Tonin is a neurotransmitter, a chemical that is used to send messages to other nerves. Serotonin is very important for

regulating mood. Low levels of serotonin are associated with lower moods, and higher levels can be associated with better moods and decreased "quarrelsome" behaviours.[28] This is why Sarah is often referred to as the "happy hormone."

SSRIs manage, through medical magic, to block the reabsorption of this chemical, leading to its lingering around the body in higher concentrations. Unsurprisingly, having a happy hormone in higher concentrations seems to be a good thing for those who suffer from PMDD! About 60–70% of women with PMDD will benefit from SSRIs, and they seem to work faster in women with PMDD than in those who don't have PMDD.

The effectiveness of these drugs will vary between the people who take them, so the only way to truly know how effective they will be is to give them a try (under the supervision and on the recommendation of a competent specialist medical professional).

For us, the SSRIs were a game changer. It was the first intervention that had some palpable benefit. I would say that my wife taking these medications improved *my* life's wellbeing by 50%. The symptoms were still there, but in a diminished form.

Some observations of our own experience (this may not be the case with your partners):

- We did find that if my wife forgot to take it or ran out of medication, then later that day or for the next couple of days, the risk of acute PMDD symptoms was very high. She didn't have to tell me when medication was missed, as the change in mood and flare-up in PMDD symptoms did the explaining.
- My wife would occasionally doubt that she had PMDD, believing that it was all in her head or that she could conquer it using willpower alone and decide not to take the SSRIs. When my wife would inform me that she had decided to stop taking her medication (sometimes she didn't inform me), a chill would be sent down my spine as I knew

---

[28] How to increase serotonin in the human brain without drugs - PMC
https://www.ncbi.nlm.nih.gov/pmc/articles/PMC2077351/#r39-1

what the next few days might be like. Sometimes my wife would stop taking the medication due to side effects too.

Oral Contraceptives

Another medication used can be oral contraceptives. We found these helped reduce the symptoms of PMDD maybe a little, but the side effects were very significant for us, and we went through two different types of contraceptives before moving onto other treatments.

Further Treatments

I am not going to cover the following treatments, as there are much better and more qualified resources available online and better framed by your treating physician. Again, please look at https://iapmd.org/treatment-options if you really want a comprehensive overview of medications and treatment options. IAPMD published a comprehensive e-book of these options which I would highly recommend.

Hormone Replacement Therapy, intrauterine devices (commonly known as the coil), and GnRH agonists are all some of the options that your doctor might explore, including, as a last resort, surgery.

I am not going to cover holistic therapies, more fringe self-medication treatments like CBD oil, or more exploratory, fringe treatments like microdosing with psilocybin. There just isn't enough evidence for me to dedicate time to exploring them. If there isn't enough evidence, we can't be confident in their safety, though it is important to point out that some women will have success with these non-conventional approaches.

I think it would be useful to give some account of our experience with surgery, and it seems to be a topic of interest amongst sufferers and partners alike, so I will dedicate a little of the book to this.

Surgery

I can fit a whole Wagon Wheel (a large British chocolate biscuit!) in one mouthful, and while it is hard to speak or breathe during my display of this envious talent, it is still less of a mouthful than trying to say '*full hysterectomy and bilateral salpingo-oophorectomy'* in one go. For the sake of brevity, I will just refer to the aforementioned phrase as 'surgery'. The surgery refers to the complete removal of the uterus, fallopian tubes, and ovaries. It is important that the ovaries are removed too because they produce sex hormones, the very things responsible for triggering PMDD.

Our experience with my wife having a full hysterectomy and oophorectomy was life changing.

I am naturally built as quite a resilient person; it's not something I can take credit for, as it has always been my disposition. But in the year before my wife had her hysterectomy, the toll and strain of caring for her and our four children, one of whom has special needs, was exhausting. I work as a medical professional, and it can be quite intense. Normally, between cycles, I would take time to reboot and rebuild. However, prior to her surgery, my wife was fitted with a hormonal intrauterine device (AKA an IUD, or the coil) that seemed to just bring her into a continuous state of depression and lethargy. There was no recovery time between cycles, as there was no cycle, and it seemed that if happiness was in our home, my wife couldn't find it.

It felt like rock bottom, and I wondered if I could keep going at this level.

At our review appointment with the specialist doctor, we spoke openly with her about the current situation. By this stage, it had been seven years of trialling different interventions and medications; we were both exhausted and a mess. We had children and were not planning on having any more, and we had talked about surgery as something that we would be willing to beg for.

She sat quietly listening to us, and after hearing us out, she paused for a moment and then carefully reached into her desk drawer and pulled out a diary. She said, "When do you want the surgery?" It was like being hit with a stun gun. We were shocked. We presumed that we would have to go through more trials of different interventions. We leapt at the chance. We had already spent months or even years talking about it as an option, and though it was invasive and irreversible, it felt like the right thing to do.

After my wife had surgery, I could describe her as effectively cured of a monthly cyclical torture. Prior to the surgery, my wife and I had developed really good communication around how she was feeling. The sharp edge of PMDD had been blunted somewhat. My wife had also developed a great deal of introspection around her condition, and we felt like we had taken as much control as we possibly could, but the symptoms were still so extreme that we could not navigate them. Our level of management of PMDD was like flowing down river rapids in a raft and learning how to steer a little and control the direction, but it didn't change the fact that we were hurtling down a raging river. It was helpful to have the ability to steer away from the most dangerous places and anticipate the most difficult segments of the river. However, we were always in survival mode, and it was still perilous.

After the surgery, life felt like the rapids suddenly changed from a risky, high-pressure, high-stakes journey to a relaxing float down a slow, wide river. Surgery was such a sudden and major thing for us. It made me recognise a few things. It is now beyond a doubt just how little cognitive control she had over the symptoms of PMDD.

For the first year or so, there were random bouts of short-lived PMDD-like behaviour, since my wife was taking hormone replacement therapy (HRT). HRT is usually prescribed, as the sex hormones play important roles in protecting the body against things like osteoporosis (weakening of the bones) that can happen after menopause.

Remember that someone who has PMDD is **hypersensitive to hormonal fluctuations,** and fluctuations can still cause some symptoms. These "flare-ups" we called them, usually occurred if my wife had forgotten to take the medication, or the patch that delivered the oestrogen came off and wasn't replaced quickly, or sometimes they just seemed to happen randomly (stress!). However, this was a walk in the park compared with full-on PMDD. So after surgery, I think it's fair to expect some bumps in the road, but overall, it was amazing.

There are some things to consider post-surgery, like the ongoing balancing act of getting the right HRT and finding the dosage and method of intake (tablets, patches, etc.) which can induce varying levels of PMDD symptoms, and some may struggle with this more than others. These things are important, and they can still interfere significantly with life, but they weren't in the same league for us as PMDD.

It made me reflect again and again on how much PMDD is a life-altering condition. When you are living with PMDD, you adapt to it, and your life becomes adjusted to its rhythm. They say the best way to really see the effect of something is to take it away, and so, following my wife's surgery, I was able to see from a clear vantage point how much it had dominated our lives. When my wife and I discuss or think back on PMDD, we shudder at how extreme things were. We give each other the same type of glance that says, *'That was intense'*.

PMDD can define people's occupation, relationship status, personal finances, physical health and mental health. The reach and impact of PMDD are so extensive that it only seems natural that PMDD should be the type of condition EVERYONE should know about. If it can give such severe symptoms to up to 5% of women, then how can it be that it is so unknown?

2

RELATIONSHIPS

The Four Pillars

In the 1960s, the CIA[29] concocted a cunning plan to spy on Russia called Operation Acoustic Kitty. Complex surgery was performed on a cat to implant a microphone into its ear. The cat would also have a small radio transmitter placed at the base of the skull along with a battery stored under its fur. The project took years to complete, and the cat was to be used to listen in on conversations outside the Russian Embassy in Washington DC.

The project cost twenty million dollars and was a dismal failure and shut down. Why? Anyone who has any experience with cats will know that they do what they want and go where they want. You cannot control a cat. A cat can't be trained. No -one had really considered if the cat would be obedient. How embarrassing.

The fundamentals of the mission just hadn't been considered.

We can get caught up in trying new systems, techniques, medications with PMDD that we overlook the fundamentals aspects of relationships. In the next section I would like to cover some fundamental principles that are necessary for a relationship with someone with PMDD.

I live next to a wonderful cathedral in Durham. Built in 1133, it is one of the finest examples of architecture from that era and took forty years to construct. Buildings like that remind me of relationships. It takes time, patience, and planning to make them a success. They also need to be structurally sound to withstand the extremes.
Your relationship is similar, it needs to have a secure enough foundation of trust, commitment, love, kindness for it to function. However, there are some additional PMDD specific principles need implementation. These are the *four pillars* that are built upon those foundations to protect against the extremes of PMDD. These are:

---

[29] https://en.wikipedia.org/wiki/Acoustic_Kitty

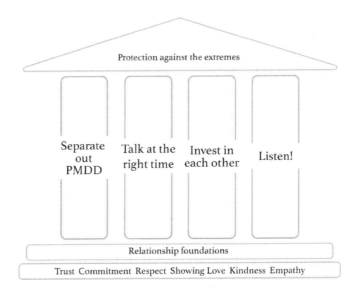

I can't emphasise enough the importance of having strong fundamentals in a relationship. Having PMDD in a relationship is like having open heart surgery every month; *you must go into it healthy so you can come out alive on the other side.*

Surgeons prefer treating a fit and healthy patient who is free from other diseases. They have the best chances of survival and recover faster. The healthier the relationship *going into* the luteal phase, the better chances you have at survival, and the quicker you will *both recover.*

The stronger[30] the relationship you both have together, the less of a destructive influence PMDD has. PMDD is like a tandem bike, you have to ride it together. If you are going to get through it successfully, both parties have to work together in unison against that common enemy: PMDD.

---

[30] The Gottman Institute as a great place to delve more into relationship fundamentals. Start with the Four Horsemen. www.gottman.com

Later in the book, there is a chapter devoted to those whose partners have PMDD who are not engaged in treatment or denying the diagnosis. I describe some methods that may be helpful in working with your partner to seek treatment. You can't really deal with any problem properly until it is properly acknowledged, and that is the point of that chapter: to help you and your partner isolate the entity of PMDD and the impact it has on each of you.

You, Me and PMDD

Separating out PMDD from your partner.

There are three entities in your relationship. You, your partner, and PMDD.

Like something out of a horror movie, its presence is haunting, lingering, and pervasive.

PMDD: It's the dementor in the corner of your room, its silent presence casting its shadow over your daily decisions. It's there from the moment you wake until you go to sleep. It's there when you are doing your shopping, making toast, or brushing your teeth. It's there when you chat, reminisce, or argue with your partner. Like a dark spectre, an ominous mass, it follows you both, emanating its influence.

It's not just You and Me; it's 'You, Me, *and PMDD.*'

Of course, you can ignore it and hope PMDD will go away; you can pretend it's *not there.* But regardless, it is still there. The more you pretend it isn't there, the more powerful PMDD gets.

You see, both of you already have independent relationships with PMDD; it already influences *each* of you in *different ways.*

PMDD can change the way you talk, listen, and touch each other. It can change the way you view your relationship in the short and long term. The quality and success of your relationship may depend on the unique relationship each of you has with PMDD. How do you interact with it? Do you ignore it? Do you fight it? Do you taunt it? Do you hide from it? Does it frame your life's experiences or expectations? Do you feed it? Or is it feeding you or your partner resentment and bitterness? Does it feed your partner's shame and guilt?

Once you are better able to differentiate the condition from the rest of the person, it can help you cope, but how can you actually isolate PMDD from your partner?

1. **Training, tracking, time & practice.** Being able to separate out PMDD from your partner really does take time and practice. It takes years tracking of cycles in a variety of situations to identify what is PMDD and how it is different to your partner's true character or any underlying relationship issues. If you think you have this wired after a few months, you are wrong.
2. **Understand what PMDD is and what it is like to have it.** We have already discussed how important it is to really get your head around PMDD, to listen and to understand. You aren't going to spot a whale on a whale watching trip if you don't know what a whale looks like.
3. **Use reference points.** Is the behaviour consistent with your partners ideals, values and beliefs. Is it contradictory to previous statements? Is this behaviour self-destructive? Do these seem like rational, reasonable and logical behaviours?
4. **Physical symptoms** may occur at the same time as psychiatric symptoms. Physical symptoms are easier to define and identify and can act as a prompt to know when your partner might be expressing behaviour related with PMDD. e.g. craving for sugar, breast tenderness, lethargy, bloating.
5. **Duration** of the behaviour. Does it match up to the PMDD cycle? Real problems and issues don't just disappear. If the belief, action or desire is persistent in its duration throughout several cycles it might not be PMDD related.
6. **Intensity.** There is an intensity with PMDD like behaviour, an urgency. Things that need solving *right now*. Look out for sudden peaks of intensity.

It can be an out of body experience for those with PMDD. My wife recounted that whilst experiencing intense rage, she could see what PMDD was making her do but could not stop it from happening. Terrifying.

Some of those with the condition have come to name their alter-ego. "Smeagol" "She-hulk" "Hagatha Christie" and "Lady Wolf-Bitch" are some names that those with PMDD have given to their PMDD.[31]

You might ask yourself, "Why can't she just get a hold of herself?" "Why can't she snap herself out of it?" Such instinctive responses may feel natural, but they do not take into account the complexity of the behavioural substructure. Consider the complexity of a normal, healthy individual and then add in a pathological neurological condition like PMDD. You can understand why someone can't just "think their way out of it" alone. *It is like asking a person in a wheelchair to stand up and run.*

Trying to cure PMDD with willpower alone is like trying to dam a river with one stone.

Will that stone help?

Yes, but more are needed!

Therapy has been shown to be effective in reducing the symptoms associated with PMDD and is worth doing. One stone won't dam a river, but each intervention is important and significant in its own right.

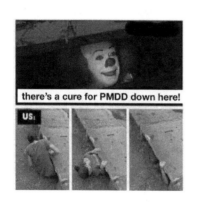

there's a cure for PMDD down here!

US.

You can't change a fundamentally physiological condition purely through psychological means alone. I am sceptical of the overselling of psychological therapies as a singular complete fix for PMDD, especially where "cures" are promised along with "rapid results." Beware of PMDD clickbait cures. Psychological therapies, in my opinion, are essential in helping patients manage the condition, but they aren't the PMDD panacea.

---

[31] Courtesy of subreddit r/PMDD

I can speak from my own experience when I say that after my wife had her hysterectomy, I realised just how little control she had prior. I knew PMDD was responsible for so much of her behaviour during that time, but I must admit I was astonished at how much of that anger and discontent left along with her uterus and ovaries.

Once you differentiate the person from the condition, you start to be able to see what behaviour is more of a direct result of the PMDD. At least PMDD is helpful in having a clearly defined pattern, usually starting a week or two before the period. If you find that symptoms persist through the whole month, this can be due to medication or perhaps another co-morbid condition (e.g., bipolar disorder, depression, anxiety) expressing itself as a a Premenstrual Exacerbation. It may be slightly easier to not take things personally when you recognise the behaviour directed at you is characteristically PMDD luteal phase behaviour. Just as people are innocent until proven guilty, it is proper that due diligence be followed to establish if there is a good reason behind the behaviour rather than casting it off as personality or bad behaviour. It is about not jumping to conclusions.

As time went on, I was able to define more and more what was PMDD and what was just part of my wife's personality. I must admit it was easier for me because my wife is inherently the opposite of the PMDD symptoms she showed. There was a real Jekyll and Hyde dynamic. The more cognitive separation of PMDD that occurs, the more likely you are to see the following benefits:

- *Reduce the shame or guilt of PMDD.* Your partner will feel wracked with guilt for their behaviour. PMDD sufferers can't switch off symptoms. Mask them? Sure. Being able to recognise the lack of control a sufferer has over these symptoms is liberating for both partners. The guilt adds to stress and the stress exacerbates PMDD symptoms.

- *More able to talk to others about it.* You may find that both you and your partner feel more comfortable talking to others about it. The more people that understand the cyclical hardship that families may go through, the better.

- *Examine and review more objectively.* When you and your partner review PMDD episodes during the follicular phase, you may find the heat taken out of the conversations as you both separate the condition from the person. You and your partner may feel more comfortable expressing feelings as it is safer. It turns what could be an emotional shouting match into a considerate, candid open discussion filled with PMDD revelatory experiences.

- *Hurt reduces.* PMDD inflates everyday minor problems into overwhelming, life changing problems. What she says about you, might only represent a very, very small amount of how she feels really. Though unkind words and behaviour will still hurt, the reason she says them is because she is ill. It doesn't represent who she really is, *she* is the person filled with regret for the words spoken after the PMDD subsides. However, many sufferers feel unable to raise the subject again out of embarrassment, shame, or in some cases they genuinely do not remember.

Practically, separating the condition from the person helps you not take things as personally, removes shame from the condition, makes you more able to talk to others about it and look at things more objectively.

Talk at the right time.

Try to avoid discussing PMDD issues during the luteal phase. When you are in a burning building, it is not the time to have a fire safety discussion. When you are on a sinking ship, it's not the time to discuss why it's sinking. You can't negotiate when you are under heavy machine-gun fire. Talking has to be done at the right time to be effective. I *can't emphasise this enough.* So many times, I initiated 'discussions' that turned into arguments. It was against my better judgement, and it never ended well.

The most meaningful, reflective discussions happen on your partner's terms, naturally, when they are in the right place mentally.

"When me and my partner started working with expressing and talking with radical honesty, she was pretty amazed that you can actually talk about pretty difficult stuff without things blowing up. She was so used to that happening in the past. And that history of chaos creates a very deep insecurity, and I think my partner plays that out as a kind of anticipation that she WILL be rejected."

A partner - PMDD support group

Yes, after menstruation is the time to talk and reflect. As tempting as it might be, you do not want to try and chat about PMDD during the luteal phase. It's a trap! You can very easily get drawn into The Doom Loop of false narratives, paranoia, exacerbated relationship issues and back breaking mental gymnastics. These complexities can't be effectively dealt with through the lens of the luteal phase.

There may be occasions where you feel your partner is enticing you into a loaded discussion. *How do you avoid being drawn in while at the same time not ignoring your partner or invalidating their concerns?*

There may be considerable pressure on you to respond or make a decision. One solution may come from an unlikely source; watching politicians being interviewed. They are slick masters of evasiveness. If you want a lesson on how to avoid giving a definitive answer, delay, distract while still seeming to satisfy the demands of hungry journalists, then politicians are the greatest example. The difference is you aren't a politician, and you care about your partner and their feelings. I found affirmative statements like the following helped:

"I love you, and I can see this is important to you right now, but I want to think things over a bit so I can answer you properly. Can we talk about this later on?"

"You have made your point, and I am trying to understand why you feel this way. I really think I will need more time to consider the points you have made."

If there are times when whatever you say is used against you and no matter what you say or do will appease PMDD. Take the Ronan Keating approach, by using the line out his hit song, "You Say It Best, When you Say Nothing At All"

First rule of PMDD Fight Club is you do not talk about PMDD during Luteal Fight time.

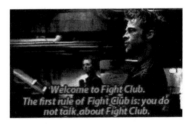

Does your partner mean what is said in the heat of the luteal phase?

Yes. Your partner normally means what they say, *at that moment.*

Your partner may say things that are out of character. The comments may not feel representative of their normal core values or beliefs. Your partner may say things about you that don't reflect how they normally speak about you or the relationship. Regardless, at that moment, your partner still normally means what they say. However, there are many times where after the period arrives there is a clarity of thought that can occur and *some* things that were important, aren't as important anymore. That is why many of those with PMDD give themselves a rule...

"No big decisions in the premenstrual phase."

How do you know your partner's true position? It isn't easy. If the opinion stays consistent through the whole cycle and is reflective of past behaviour, then this is a good indication. This comment by a partner on a PMDD forum provides some guidance.

"The way I look at it is yes, she absolutely means the things she says when she says them, but she's not herself when she says them. If those feelings persist over time (and by that I mean that they don't subside with the PMDD, because she will absolutely say them again during a future episode), then you can begin to question whether that's how she truly feels. But if she only says these things at flashpoints in her cycle, then try not to take them personally. Once you can divorce the PMDD version of your partner from the real version, who you know and love and who loves you back, it's much easier (but still difficult!) to put those comments in context."

Post-luteal blues

You would think you would be throwing down the red carpet and popping champagne to welcome the non-PMDD partner back like a war hero. However, there are two things to consider:

1. It might not be over yet. Some PMDD symptoms can last for a few of days after the period arrives.

"Try not to remind her of things she said in her right mind when she's in her wrong mind. It will only inflame things and make her feel like her present feelings are being invalidated. All of the things she said about loving you and trusting you and wanting to build a family with you are true. But when the hormones take over, her world is crumbling around her and she won't feel any of those things. If you can keep the faith and limit the damage during episodes like this, then the partner who loves you will be waiting on the other side of it."

SP- PMDD Partner Support

2. Your partner's "switch" back to being themselves can be a sudden change. It's a psychological whiplash. It is hard as a partner to make that change so quickly. You can feel exhausted and confused. It can take time to process what might have happened in the luteal phase. It is also normal for you to feel spaced out and down while you get your head around things. Your partner might feel that you are being distant or removed. The mind takes time to process things.

It's also tempting, once the follicular phase hits, to straight away offload onto your partner all the things they might have said to you over the last week or two. It's natural that you feel like this. However, dig deep into your self-control and develop all the zen of a meditating Shaolin monk[32] to give your partner the space necessary to talk when *they are ready* during that phase and are in a good frame of mind. Just as the best parties are those that aren't planned, conversations about PMDD are the best when they happen organically. There is nothing so sweet as those moments of mutual understanding and reconcilement. Those moments are the antidote to the poison of PMDD. As pointed out previously, your partner will still be mentally recovering, processing and reconciling the luteal phase too.

---

[32] Shaolin monks are renowned for their control over their bodies and minds. One of the most elite Shaolin monks, Tai Jin who suffered from hypertrichosis (excessive body hair) was abandoned at the monastery as a baby because of his body hair. The monks raised him and trained him. He eventually dedicated himself to one form of martial art. Legend also has it that upon meeting the 12 masters of Shaolin, the boy threw a dagger into the ceiling, killing a would-be assassin. He explained to the masters that he could hear 13 people breathing, not just 12. This has nothing to do with PMDD but it felt necessary to include just because Tai Jin sounded pretty cool.

Invest in each other.

Deposits and withdrawals: keep a healthy balance.

I want you to imagine that relationships are like bank accounts; there are deposits and withdrawals. Every time your partner feels connected to or positive about you for any reason, this is a deposit in the account. However, every time your partner feels disconnected or negative towards you for any reason, it is a withdrawal.

Most relationships, we would hope, exist on the basis that each party agrees to make regular positive deposits, and though inevitably there are occasional and inadvertent small withdrawals, the bank account remains healthy and the relationship remains fulfilling and strong. Deposits may be things like: providing an act of help, a genuine compliment, spending quality time with each other, listening to each other, intimacy, laughing at each other's jokes, doing a fun activity together, or doing something new with each other. Withdrawals could be criticism (remember that rejection sensitivity dysphoria may be heightened for those with PMDD), arguments, breaches in trust, unmet expectations, not pulling your weight with housework, insensitivity, overreacting and verbal abuse.

Getting overdrawn

Problems in relationships can often begin when withdrawals become larger and more frequent than deposits, putting the relationship overdrawn and deeply in the red. This puts the short-term and long-term viability of the relationship under strain.

Imagine now, if we continue with the bank account analogy, that you have a payment called "PMDD." It's a standing order, a direct debit that comes out every month. In fact, it's more than that; its multiple payments made every day for 7–14 days every month. It is like PMDD is purposely trying to decimate your finances, empty the account of all deposits, and take your relationship to bankruptcy. For many months, it can feel like PMDD clears out almost every pound or dollar, sometimes leaving your relationship penniless and destitute. Because the payment is different each month and some months are higher than others, it is hard to budget and *anticipate* exactly what will be required. Regardless, the payment of PMDD becomes due, and it puts strain on the relationship.

While you don't have control over this withdrawal, *you do have some control over how many deposits are made beforehand.* The more deposits that are made into the relationship, the healthier you can keep the balance, and the harder it is to reach absolute rock bottom or a crisis point. Make a list of the things your partner enjoys. Take the time to embrace the follicular phase. Try to make those emotional investments.

Unfortunately, with PMDD, no matter what you do, you may find that despite your best efforts, at least temporarily, the balance of your account seems to be completely cleared out. Investing more proactively in the relationship isn't prophylaxis against PMDD, but it does take the edge off the severity and reduce the risk of a particularly severe cycle. In those moments, try to remember that **it is just temporary**. Things *should* return gradually after the luteal phase completes.

Make the most of the follicular phase.

Having a partner with PMDD also means you have *less time* to make those positive contributions to a relationship, having only two or three weeks rather than four. The contributions you make are more critical and need to last longer. You can't cruise through a relationship with someone with PMDD. Relationships with PMDD are grindingly hard work; they are at the coalface. If you are seeking out those diamonds among the rocks. The follicular phase is time to strengthen your relationship.

Build on the simple fundamentals.

You will remember the diagram below from earlier in the book, showing the four pillars built on the foundation of relationship fundamentals.
The foundations of any relationship are trust, commitment, respect and expressions of love.

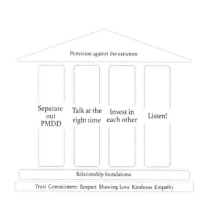

Contributions of kindness, forgiveness, and understanding are so valuable, as is the power to admit when you are wrong. Sometimes withholding anger or a sarcastic comment might be all you can muster, but it is a deposit, nonetheless. Thoughtfulness, compliments, and quality time connect people together. Find the things, hobbies, and subjects that you both enjoy talking about and talk more about them. Do new things together, build a culture of gratitude.

You are not solely responsible for the success of the relationship.

You should expect that if you are both working collaboratively together that those foundational relationship principles are a joint venture. It's about each of you reciprocating positive behaviours the best you can.

Your partner should be actively contributing to the relationship, depending on how well they are doing. If you are at the stage where you can both sit down and make a plan, don't just plan the luteal phase; plan during the follicular phase to do some enjoyable things together.

Regardless of your partner's engagement, start by making these deposits unconditional – you don't expect anything back, and with time and luck, your partner will reciprocate. That reciprocation by your partner is the interest on your deposits. It is the positive reinforcement of positive actions, building rather than destroying.

These foundational behaviours build trust and safety and open the door for vulnerable honest conversations. What I am recommending is hard, but it is also life-enhancing.

What not to do

If you want to wipe out your emotional bank account with your partner, then constantly keep telling her how awful she is to you and telling her to stop it. *She can't*; it's not that simple. The weight of the guilt brings her down further, along with her self-worth and dignity, and it decays your relationship.

Heaping guilt on your partner is like putting holes in a boat that is already sinking; it adds suffering to someone who is already suffering. Whilst destructive behaviours toward you need to be addressed directly, guilting someone when they are vulnerable is not constructive. It can also heighten the risk of harm to them.

Compounding interest.

In investing terms, compound interest is the interest you earn on your interest. Over time, the accumulation of this interest helps form a nest egg of wealth. The investments you make in the relationship are self-reinforcing and self-reinvesting; they will gain "interest," for example, as your partner feels the relationship improving and the trust deepening, there is an increased likelihood that you can share the ways the condition might impact you. Your experience in the relationship is just as important and valid as your partner's. It is easy for your views and feelings to be lost or overlooked as the symptoms of PMDD become overwhelming. Each of us carries around too much guilt about letting other people down. *We can't control what other people expect of us; we can only control what we expect of ourselves.* Perhaps the most important promises we make are the ones where we promise to be "our best selves."

As you build your partner up, there will hopefully be a reduction in their self-loathing, shame, and guilt. The reduction of these toxic traits should be liberating and may open the door for your partner to pursue the goals they have in life.

As time went on for me and my wife, we both gained a very open understanding of PMDD and working on it together strengthened us. We knew what it looked like, where it liked to pop up, and how it affected both of us. We knew the enemies' game plan. PMDD forced us into a state of heightened communication with deeper patience, trust, and mutual support, and as paradoxical as it seems, we are stronger together because of PMDD. Working together was an extreme exercise in patience, understanding one another, and suffering in our own way. Nothing brings people together like a common enemy! Remember that progress is rarely visible immediately; it manifests itself over a lifetime and is best spotted when you look back over your shoulder.

When you are at the stage where there is openness and recognition of the condition, you can move on to a collaborative approach and develop a care plan.

Recognise hidden achievements.

Your partner is not like others who do not experience PMDD. Your partner's achievements will have come at a greater effort and cost than those of most of their peers. They're a secret superhero, with their heroic acts largely unrecognised in public, with only their inner circle knowing their successes. Your partner is strong. Who else has to work so hard just to get through the day and stay alive? Never mind the pressures of work, family, promotions, or volunteering. Far from being "weak" and "helpless," they are warriors and made of solid metal. Celebrate their achievements, no matter how small they may seem to others.

I should also note that it takes incredible mental and emotional fortitude to be the partner of someone who has PMDD. There is nothing easy about it, and everything is hard. I appreciate what it sometimes takes to "just keep going." The strength to love someone in the face of such cyclical bitterness, anger, and sometimes maltreatment is noble. I recognise that for some, especially those with additional life stresses and difficulties, managing PMDD may be too much of a challenge. If you are in a relationship that is already vastly withdrawn, you should ask yourself, "Is it possible that I can rebuild it?" People can judge a person by the car they drive, the house they own, and how they look. I can't help feeling the pinnacle of human achievement is found in patience and unconditional love towards our fellow beings within the walls of our own homes.

It is going to take the best of you to help her

Listening.

"When people share their problems, they're not always looking for solutions. They are often seeking support.
Sharing bad news may not make them feel better, but it does bring you closer.

The most basic form of compassion is not alleviating distress. It's acknowledging distress."

Adam Grant

Consider the account below from Stephen Covey,[33]

"I was riding a subway one Sunday morning in New York. People were sitting quietly – some reading newspapers, some lost in thought, some resting with their eyes closed. It was a calm, peaceful scene. Then suddenly, a man and his children entered the subway car. The children were so loud and rambunctious that instantly the whole climate changed.

"The man sat down next to me and closed his eyes, apparently oblivious to the situation. The children were yelling back and forth, throwing things, and even grabbing people's papers. It was very disturbing. And yet, the man sitting next to me did nothing.

"It was difficult not to feel irritated. I could not believe that he could be so insensitive as to let his children run wild like that and do nothing about it, taking no responsibility at all. It was easy to see that everyone else on the subway felt irritated, too. So finally, with what I felt was unusual patience and restraint, I turned to him and said, "Sir, your children are really disturbing a lot of people. I wonder if you couldn't control them a little more?" The man lifted his gaze as if to come to a consciousness of the

---

[33] Seven Habits of Highly Effective People. S Covey

situation for the first time and said softly, "Oh, you're right. I guess I should do something about it. We just came from the hospital where their mother died about an hour ago. I don't know what to think, and I guess they don't know how to handle it either."

"Can you imagine what I felt at that moment? My paradigm shifted. Suddenly I saw things differently, I felt differently and I behaved differently. My irritation vanished. I didn't have to worry about controlling my attitude or my behaviour; my heart was filled with the man's pain. Feelings of sympathy and compassion flowed freely. "Your wife just died? Oh, I'm so sorry. Can you tell me about it? What can I do to help?" Everything changed in an instant."

I read this account in Stephen Covey's book "The 7 Habits of Highly Effective People" when I was in my late teens, and it stuck with me. There are reasons why people behave in a certain way. People act on a prompt or motivation, and when we understand what those prompts are, we understand the person better.

We all recognise that we could be that person on the subway. Dr Covey's feelings of irritation and anger changed to sympathy and compassion just because he understood a bit more about a person's circumstances. So it is with PMDD.

Sometimes in my professional job I see parents who bring their small child into the clinic and they say, "My son has had some toothache; we think he is just putting it on a bit for attention, but we just want to get it checked." I then examine the child and identify a painful infection that the child has been self-managing for some time. I often wonder how many behavioural issues such as tantrums, unwillingness to eat food, and lack of concentration could have been influenced by such a simple thing as toothache.

You can see the shift in attitude that occurs as I explain the diagnosis to the parents. How they wished they had listened to the child earlier on. There is a paradigm shift from blaming the child as just "attention seeking" to understanding *why*. When you explore why, you find reasons rather than excuses.

I have often thought, "Who actually wants to be a nasty person?" Hardly anyone at all. It is a lazy shortcut to label someone as indolent, rude, or crazy without taking the time, patience, and empathy to understand them. Behind every behaviour is a *reason*. Even the most bizarre behaviour may have equally bizarre underlying reasoning![34]

My day-to-day learning with PMDD over the years and watching my wife struggle convinced me that she had almost no control over her mood or behaviour during the depths of PMDD. This was confirmed by the massive change post-surgery. It was satisfying to see that most of the negatively impacting behaviours I witnessed were due to PMDD. If I had spent the time blaming her rather than trying to understand PMDD, then I wouldn't have gotten the chance to enjoy the happy and healthy relationship we have now.

Be compassionate, listen to your partner. Genuinely try to understand what your partner is feeling and going through and develop deep empathy for what she is experiencing. Try to imagine what it is like to have your world fall apart every month. Imagine the hopeless depressive feelings, crippling anxiety, and relentless rage. Imagine trying to cope with the strains of life and the expectations of others at work, in family, and with your kids when the reality is that you're secretly falling apart and just trying to stay alive. Imagine not having a partner who understands what you are going through.

While the above paragraph aptly describes what a PMDD sufferer will experience, you might have read it and identified with some of the same feelings: "That is what it is like for me as a partner." You might have more in common with your partner during this time than you think!

The risk of relationship issues is higher because both people are in a bad place. The contagion of PMDD is real. Both of you feed off the negative energy.

---

[34] Or perhaps a completely reasonable reason!

When a person acts hurt, they are acting out how they feel. Have you ever had an argument where it felt like both you and your partner were shouting at each other the same message? "I AM HURTING!" "YOU DON'T UNDERSTAND!". This level of communication is a hot mess. No one is listening because they are so desperate to be understood.

Where there is no listening, there will be no learning. If your partner can't listen, then you might have to try and be the "de-escalator" and take the initiative to create the space and start listening; be the one to break the cycle.

Be the first to listen.

Despite the turmoil and the breadth of what you must deal with, you might need to put your own difficulties to one side just **temporarily**. Do this so you can spend some time trying to understand her. It is incredibly hard to put to one side, even just temporarily, the hurt, pain, and exhaustion you might be experiencing, but looking beyond our own feelings and experiences is the most superhuman thing you can possibly do. Dealing with PMDD is not one person's sole responsibility in the relationship; it is each person's responsibility to give 100 percent of *what they can*. That is a true partnership. You can't really know or control what percentage effort your partner will be putting in (remember capacity inflates/deflates), but *you can* control what effort you make.

Where possible, during the non-PMDD phase. Ask questions:

"What is it like when you experience PMDD? How does it feel?"

"What are some things I do that help you?"

"What things do I do that wind you up or make things worse?"

"What things help you feel better during that time?"

"What kind of thoughts come into your mind?"

"Who do you feel understands you?"

"What do you want to achieve that you struggle to do?"

"How do you view me during the luteal phase?"

"What symptom do you find the most overpowering?"

"What makes your struggle harder?"

A practical example of the little things that come from listening to your partner is as follows: when my wife was having an acute PMDD episode, she would be incredibly upset, perhaps angry. I could see the way she was feeling and felt I had to be by her side to comfort her during this time. Maybe by sitting close to her with my arm around her, just listening to her, or expressing how much I care for her. This is conventionally what you would expect comfort to look like, but for my wife, during those acute episodes, she genuinely wanted to be on her own. It was hard for me to walk away, and I felt like I was deserting her in her moment of need, and sometimes I worried for her physical safety. Space was what she wanted and what was best for her. Trying to maintain social interactions or look after someone else's feelings when you are struggling to cope with your own emotions sometimes makes you feel emotionally overextended. As I explored this, I recognised the same feeling. When I have experienced the death of a loved one or intense grief, I have found it overwhelming and easier to manage if I am alone. When my wife was saying, "Leave me alone," she meant it. She was saying, "I can't cope with anything, including you. Please give me space."

Don't underestimate how powerful listening is. As your partner talks, don't interrupt; just ask questions about what she means, clarify the points she is making, and restate back to her "So you mean you feel like...?" This is all so you can really understand her headspace. Ultimately, first seek to understand her, so you can be understood later.

Is it possible to understand too far? No. Is it being 'too nice'? No. Understanding someone isn't synonymous with accepting everything they do or allowing unhealthy behaviours towards you.

Another practical example: it's tempting to believe that your partner doesn't want your love because they might not enjoy being touched or hugged. However, they absolutely do want your love – oftentimes, they just need it to be expressed differently. It took me a while to discover this, and perhaps I would have learned it quicker if I had just listened and *believed*. I didn't have to take things personally. It was a burden I didn't need to have. I learned that I could express my love verbally or in other ways than just physically: through a smile, a note. If your partner doesn't want to be touched, don't see it as a rejection.

During the *luteal* phase, your approach will be different. During hard times, people don't want to be told, "Look on the bright side." They want to know that you are on *their side*.

Even if you can't help them feel better, you can help them feel understood. It's not about cheering up your partner; it's more about showing up and *just being there*.

Just being there is a demonstration of love. Emphasise how much you recognise the hurt she is going through and how much you want to support her. Show empathy, not sympathy.[35] There may be times in the follicular phase when she feels comfortable talking about what it is like to be in the luteal phase. Seize these moments and don't waste them.

Don't put rocks in your backpack.

I remember once going hiking with a friend. I noticed he was lagging behind and really seemed to be struggling not far into the hike. He was slower, and we would have to keep stopping. It was frustrating, as we needed to be at a certain point by a certain time before dark to set up camp. I didn't understand why he was so slow; after all, we were at the same level of fitness. At one point, we stopped. As he sat exhausted, I picked up the slumped backpack that lay beside him. It was so heavy! His food supplies consisted of a multitude of canned foods. I was really into hiking, and I always packed light. almost to the point where I would saw off the handle of the toothbrush to ensure that the cumulative weight would be kept to a minimum. No wonder it was so difficult for him. I think there are two PMDD lessons here.

---

35 Sympathy vs Empathy https://www.youtube.com/watch?v=KZBTYViDPlQ

1. **I didn't understand why things were so hard for him until I started to carry what he was carrying.** Once I felt the weight of what he was experiencing, the burden he was experiencing was clear. So it is with your partner. Once you understand what your partner is dealing with, you can start to work constructively.

2. **Don't make your PMDD journey harder by filling up your "mental rucksack" with stuff that isn't necessary.** Let the little things go, so you can concentrate on the bigger, more important things. They aren't worth the fight to carry them. It may be that you are carrying a heavy mental load and you need a professional to talk to. Therapy is for everyone.

Read the Room

While the principles of listening, being supportive, and being compassionate don't change, the methodology you adopt should change depending on where your partner is in their cycle.

The luteal phase is when you try to **offset some of the symptoms of PMDD** – anger, anxiety, stress and depression. Your role is to make sure the negative things aren't as negative as they could be.[36] It's *damage limitation.*

In the example I gave earlier on in the book, it's the equivalent of just buying a new sandwich for your partner or finding the hotel as quickly as you can.

Approaching the different menstrual phases

Luteal	Follicular
Short term **Symptom Management**	*Long-term* **Strategic Investment and Leadership**
• Employ coping strategies • Damage limitation • Keeping everybody safe • Providing practical care to your partner (food, space, cleaning) • Self-care • Finding space and strength to carry on • Affirming love through word or deed • Comfortable surroundings • Reducing expectations	• Rebuilding and reinvigorating • Affirming relationship foundations • Re-evaluating approaches and behaviours during luteal phase • Reflection • Engaging with treatment options • Liaising and advocating for your partner with medical practitioners • Boundary setting • Care planning

---

[36] Again, remember you are not the cause of PMDD.

There is a stressful work deadline for your partner and it's exacerbating their symptoms. The PMDD is directing the dysphoria toward you verbally. The things that are said are personal and hurtful. Of course, it's not fair to you. It is perfectly natural for you to feel angry and defensive at the behaviour and blame PMDD. In your anger, you tell her that her PMDD is bad and it's not your fault that the project deadline is stressing her out (which is the truth). How productive is this approach? Yes, there is a momentary cathartic release in saying out loud the true situation; however, in my experience, it escalates the situation. Think of the previous example of the "sandwich drop." Manage the symptoms in the short term.

When you have PMDD but still try to take a vacation

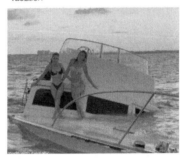

Can you find a constructive way to help? e.g. help her with the deadline? Remove some other obstacles that might allow her more time to work on the deadline? Your life improves when she is in a better place. Supporting someone in acute need doesn't reinforce or "enable" negative behaviour. This kind of support reinforces that you are there for her. Of course, where possible, discussions in the follicular phase could centre on how to prevent such a situation from occurring again.

Wars are won through preparation. That is why the follicular phase is all about strategy, planning, and investment. Rational, calm discussion during the follicular phase is the golden goose and is an investment that pays dividends in the long term.

When you do talk together, your goal shouldn't be to "prove she was wrong" or who was right; you should be helping to *reinforce the relationship* and helping *your partner gain as much self-insight as possible.*

Less "who is right" and more "what is right."

Self-insight leads to more self-control. That can't be rushed and must be delicate. I believe that if you truly have the best interests of your partner at heart, then a calm, empathetic discussion can be transformational. After all, how would you like to be treated?

3

THE EXTREMES OF PMDD

Rage, Anger and Meltdowns

"Before I was in a relationship, I used to experience these large blow-ups on my own and they were terrifying. But now, I usually blow up at my partner ... it normally begins because I start feeling STRONGLY about something he has or hasn't done, and I think I am in the right and that I have the ability to bring it up constructively. It's like I cannot shut my mouth. I quickly get triggered if he even so much as seems defensive, and I lose control and start escalating. PMDD seems to reduce my ability to communicate, and I feel trapped. It results in panic attack physical symptoms, wailing crying, screaming, sometimes hitting myself to the point of pain, INTENSE feelings of shame for "ruining my partner's life", suicidal urges, and a lot of yelling. It takes me about 45 minutes to a couple hours to calm down, then I have momentary relief for the rest of the evening (this normally happens in the evening or night). I also basically CANNOT calm down without reassurance and de-escalation from my partner, which is hard for him since he's been arguing back with me and is mad at me for the things I've said and he's scared of the way I am acting (I am not like this when not in luteal). I normally am EXTREMELY tired after (it's SUCH a release of energy).

I go to bed okay, but the next day I am absolutely riddled with guilt. I feel like I go through a mourning period and often times feel the most shame I could possibly feel. I see myself as completely unloveable. Thankfully, if I try very hard, I can use some cognitive skills to get me back on my feet by the end of the night. Then, the next day I wake up and it's like a fog has lifted. I always say I feel "Claritin clear" and then I start again on my two-ish weeks of being able to be my true self before ovulating."

PMDD sufferer, PMDD forum

Why rage? Why did this have to be a symptom? Why? Why? Why? Why something so destructive? Why something so damaging? Instead of rage, couldn't it have been a mildly pleasurable tingling in the fingertips or a gentle feeling of calm peacefulness? Why?

PMDD is so stupid.

Rage can be defined as *anger that is very strong or uncontrolled,* and it can be a major symptom in PMDD. It can shatter relationships, burn bridges, and provide some really awkward situations. It can do so much harm to the person experiencing PMDD, both by affecting decision-making and by becoming a source of self-shame.

Later on, I talk about meltdowns and what you might experience in the more acute phases of PMDD. In this section, I am going to talk about anger and rage, speculate about why they happen, and discuss what, if anything, we can do about them and why in particular the anger or rage might be particularly directed at you.

It's important to note that although we are going to concentrate on the rage in your partner, **the biggest challenge of living with someone who experiences intense anger is to *avoid becoming angry yourself.*** When you are feeling on edge, perhaps reaching the threshold of your tolerance, there is a temptation to "let it go" or fight fire with fire. You give in to the rising emotions and become angry yourself. As

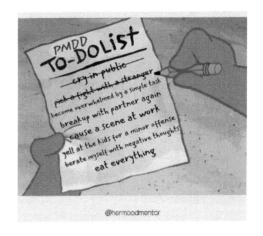

tempting as it is, try as much as you can to keep it cool. **Leave the situation if you can.** Resentment and anger are contagious, and when you act reactively, they can make you into a person you don't want to be and do things that you will regret.

What is the point of anger?[37]

Sometimes anger can also be described as "primary" or "secondary." **Primary anger** is the thing that made you angry in that moment (the stubbed toe, the flat tire) whereas **secondary anger** is "what lurks beneath"; shame, uncertainty, depressive moods, injustice, unfairness. Psychologists suspect that anger is an integral part of the natural "fight or flight" response, which means that anger has a function; it's here for a reason. *Anger is meant to protect you from danger.*

For example, when we appear angry and aggressive, we look more hostile or dangerous to a potential attacker, protecting us from further harm. Furthermore, anger plays an important role in protecting our psychological safety, which is why we can get angry when our beliefs are challenged.

For example, you spent a great deal of time on a project for work, and another colleague is very critical of the project. You feel it is unjust and unnecessarily personal, and this makes you angry.

Why?

Anger is there to protect your psychological position from threats and the threat is your own reputation, job security, ideas in the project, etc.
This anger might give you increased **short-term motivation** to deal with an imminent threat, such as confronting your work colleague, or it might give you increased **confidence in your own assertions** to argue your point. When we are angry, our self-shame and awareness of others reduces, this is your body's way of removing uncertainty in order to deal with the challenge.

Ultimately anger is about making someone feel **more powerful and less vulnerable.**

---

[37] Dr Jess Peters & IAPMD gives an excellent lecture on Rage & Anger here: https://youtu.be/VLqxb6Pc8MQ?si=bjG0Srz3T9qey69y

When someone experiences PMDD, almost everything can become a trigger. It turns normal, mundane domestic life into something intolerable. Normal, routine things that wouldn't normally bother your partner become external sources of *primary anger*. There are so many triggering *external* events because there is so much going on *internally*. PMDD is creating all sorts of internal psychological problems in the brain and so the threshold of tolerance is lowered. PMDD seems to lift the lid off the mind and pour in feelings of shame, depression, paranoia, uncertainty, sensitivity and the expectation of rejection or invalidation.

That is how PMDD seems to activate both the external and internal pathways for anger *at the same time*. That's why PMDD anger isn't just anger; it's double-whammy anger. It's a whopper.

It's rage.

The increased irritability is the "tinder," then you add in external or environmental factors as the "spark," but what really causes the fire to burn and explode are those biologically driven internal feelings of dysphoria.

Perhaps the rage is the body's way of trying to cope with these overwhelming feelings. No wonder that a simple external event like dropping a sandwich can be enough to tip the balance into a meltdown. Like a swelling dam, the rage is looking for an outlet. Something to let it all flood out. Perhaps that is why your behaviour becomes a focal point. PMDD needs something to blame.

"I won't abandon you when your PMDD acts up..."

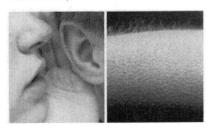

This sometimes makes the person who is experiencing PMDD attribute the rage they feel to the external trigger, when really 99% of it may come from the weight of all those awful feelings. It is no wonder that those who have PMDD may misinterpret or blame symptoms they experience on other factors.

This is the process by which PMDD inflates and exaggerates.

There might be some accompanying behaviours that get thrown in with the rage. It's a bit of a "buy one, get everything else free" scenario. These are accompanying features that sometimes come with the rage, such as heightened anxiety and paranoia with some post-rage shame.

Anger is such a strong emotion that I feel it is sometimes used by the body to hide the more vulnerable, intimate emotions. Anger is about self-protection. Maybe for your partner, anger is the better emotion to present than exposing the vulnerabilities such as shame and anxiety.

Temporary Self-Centredness or Narcissism

Everyone has the capacity to become a bit narcissistic when feeling angry or resentful, and there are reasons why this can happen. In the adrenaline rush of anger, you feel a surge of power and might feel entitled and more important than those around you—that you must take *priority*. Remember, anger's function is one of protection, and a person experiencing anger will put themselves first to protect themselves and their interests. There can be a false sense of confidence or arrogance. You might also find the anger provides re more motivation for your partner to sway the situation to become more favourable to themselves. This is all part of the prioritisation that anger can bring. Additionally, you may notice that there might be reduced empathy from your partner; they might be less likely to see things from your viewpoint. That's another reason not to argue when a situation is clouded by too much emotion.

Victim Identity

When resentment and anger are present, people might see themselves as *reacting to an unfair world* and believe they are victims. In many respects, it is true that those with PMDD are victims of an awful condition. Life hasn't been fair to them. However, what we are talking about here are specific feelings of victimhood *when the rage or the luteal hits* and how they can be misattributed.

If the person perceives themselves as a victim of *your* actions, it gives them a legitimate (as they feel at the time) reason to put themselves above you. Anger gives priority, and priority gives protection. If someone were to point out the unfair behaviour they exhibit during this time, they are likely to feel more attacked and unsafe and further reinforce that they are victims. This is one reason why challenging ideas and beliefs during the luteal phase is ill advised.

You may feel that, during the anger, the standards or expectations your partner imposes on you are unrealistic and unachievable. They might be! You might feel "damned if you do, damned if you don't." Driven by high standards of what your partner feels they should get and what other people should do for them, they may often feel disappointed and offended by you, which in turn causes more entitlement. It seems only fair, from their perspective, that they be compensated for their constant frustrations. Special consideration seems like so little to ask!
The logic follows: "It's so hard being me; I shouldn't have to do the dishes either!"

As always, it's *not quite that simple.* There is a balancing act. Special considerations **do** have to be given; the fatigue, the lethargy, the brain fog and dealing with the emotional burden of PMDD absolutely one hundred percent, do justify special consideration. This is where it can be hard to find that sweet spot of what is reasonable to expect from your partner versus what is not. It is my experience that learning this comes through listening, understanding and sharing experiences with your partner. As you plan for PMDD, you will have to agree together on some boundaries or red lines for how far special considerations should be taken into account. PMDD can be a bit like the Gas Laws[38]–the more space you allow something under pressure, the more volume it will fill.

---

[38] The Gas Laws: https://en.wikipedia.org/wiki/Gas_laws

When your partner is angry, there might be a tendency for them to attribute bad intentions, incompetence, or inadequacy to those who might disagree with them. You probably have experienced this phenomenon yourself: when you are angry and someone doesn't agree with you, you may devalue them. "They would say that ..." "They are only saying that because ..." "He isn't an expert ..."

Combine this aspect of anger with a healthy dose of rejection sensitivity, and that is why, most times, **you cannot reason your way out of rage.**

The Blame Game

When your partner is distressed, angry, or in a rage in the luteal phase, is there a tendency to blame it on you? But you know it is PMDD, so you blame it on her. Then everyone is upset.

One of the biggest problems with anger is the subsequent blaming of an uncomfortable emotional state that they experience on other (usually innocent) people or objects. The rush that comes with anger gives increased confidence. That sense of power and confidence that comes with anger feels so much better than the powerlessness and vulnerability the person might have felt before.

Whatever goes up must come down. That surge of exponential power that comes with the rage inevitably peaks and subsides into diminished energy—tired, apathetic, exhausted. And that's just the *physical* response; it does not include having to deal with the *psychological* effects of having done something while you're angry that you are later ashamed of, like hurting people you love.

The law of blame says that it eventually goes to the closest person. The PMDD-induced resentment and anger is likely to blame you for the problems of the relationship, work problems, and the price of milk—everything—and, if your partner perceives that you are to blame for everything, what motivation is there during the luteal phase to change or improve themselves in that moment? They feel they don't need changing; you do!

So, what can we do?

We can accept that negative feelings are going to come in the luteal phase regardless of your behaviour. You can't stop the tide from pushing no matter what you do. However, we can offset the rage a little by helping our partner in a few different ways.

Make the person feel safe. If anger is a response to feeling unsafe or under threat, then the antidote is making sure your partner feels *safe*, both emotionally and physically. You aren't going to rage or become abusive or violent yourself, and you aren't going to berate her for the things she does wrong. Safety is found in having a strong relationship. All the non-urgent but important work of building trust in the relationship is the foundational work for those moments.

We can try to distinguish between what are symptoms of the cycle and what are genuine, justifiable rage-inducing events, i.e. what is PMDD, and who is your partner? Once we are able to separate these entities, you can try to...

Help *your partner* distinguish between symptoms of the cycle and genuine, justifiable rage-inducing events. *Key point: this is likely a follicular phase-only activity.* Reflect together on your responses to a difficult situation. Try to be objective. Almost like sports people reviewing their plays in a match, both compassionately consider the performance and look at ways it could be improved. Avoid blaming but take ownership of what you could have done better. Again, this is probably best done in the follicular phase.

How much success have you had previously during emotionally charged arguments? Probably not much. Remember, not only is your partner angry at that moment, but they will also be in a heightened state where their brain is *expecting* rejection or invalidation and are probably more likely to interpret any behaviour by you as such.

Here is a great post by partner JK, posted on a support group.

"My partner is currently in her luteal phase and cannot see her role in the recent dispute we had (which to me, no one is truly at fault it was just an issue that spanned from the circumstances of life) where narcissistic behaviors and projection were in full effect that I stood back and said,

"'I hear your concerns and have apologized for my role in all of this but now there seems to be other things that are bothering you that I will not be addressing right now. I can sense the frustration and anger and due to that, it is raising the same sensations within me. I am not running away from the issue, I would just like for us to give it sometime until we are both in a healthier state of mind as I feel like if I do address them ... that it could just make matters worse. Please take all the time you need and I will let you know when I feel less reactive but I would like you to show me the same respect and let me know when you are ready to continue the discussion.'

"That seemed to have worked out pretty well! Though we didn't speak much for the rest of the day, she did come back later in the evening and apologized for her reactions and some of the language that was used. Recognizing her behavior and expressing that she just needs space right now.

"I don't know about anyone else but it seems like the reactive mode brings on a sense of shame in some who recognize their behaviors after the fact. I think it's important to acknowledge that and support them, letting them know that although what they said/did hurt us, that we are proud of them for acknowledging their role in what transpired and forgiving them (if you can find it in you)."

JK provides a really good way of handling a difficult situation. Be like JK. Don't say things like:

"You wouldn't say that if you weren't PMDDing" or *"Have you taken your meds?"* or *"You are being irrational."*

Though you might be correct, statements like this point the finger away from what your partner feels are the problems. In those moments, the problems she feels she is experiencing are real and disconnected from

PMDD and your redirection can cause feelings of invalidation and rejection and that *"you just don't get it."*

You will be stimulated and angry too. During the luteal phase, you might experience feelings of being misunderstood, angry, or lonely. **But you have to break the cycle of reactivity.** You might feel emotional fatigue, like you are running low on empathy, especially if kind gestures have been misinterpreted. Are you in the right frame of mind to discuss things with a cool head? Perhaps the strong feelings are spilling over into decisions.

If you feel inclined to make significant decisions whilst you are angry or finding the luteal phase difficult to bear, undertake the "self-assessment tool" below. Probably no one is going to feel like filling out a form when they are in a rage. But even just looking at the questions may prompt some self-reflection and context. This tool could be particularly useful for those with PMDD as well.

Who's gonna survive PMDD this month?

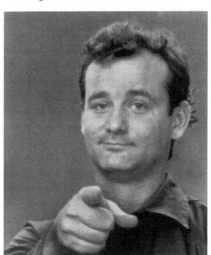

Self-Reflection Anger Tool

What is causing me to feel angry?	
Why?	
Has this caused me anger before? When?	
What am I planning on doing about it?	
Is there another side to the story I should consider? Is there another explanation I should explore?	
What questions would I need answered to make sure I am making the right decision?	
Can/should I delay action on this? **Can I slow down?** Can I take a step back?	
Is my response typical of how I would normally respond to something like this?	
Is there a calming activity I can participate in to clear my head? **Accurate perspectives empower me to make better decisions.**	
Reminders *Avoid rash behaviour even when it feels justified.* *When I am in the grip of anger,* **my judgement is clouded** *and my* **perceptions are likely distorted**	

You and your partner could consider keeping a diary of events or triggers for arguments during the luteal phase and reviewing it during the follicular phase. This exercise may help provide clarity on whether the rage was induced by cyclical symptoms or if it was an issue that needs resolving.

Controlling your own anger.

Remember, you can experience anger too. It is understandable that you will feel anger, disappointment, loneliness, and frustration. It is understandable that sometimes your anger fills to capacity and then you snap.

The anger is often less explosive and more pernicious for us as partners. It builds. Through the luteal phase, you are gradually worn down by some of the behaviours or caring responsibilities. The anger and resentment are internalised to avoid provoking a reaction from your partner. This gives more time for that secondary anger to build until the final crescendo, a dramatic "snap" of rage when you lose your temper.

You might not be handling it as well as you think you are. The 'snap' might catch you by surprise. Try to catch yourself and remove yourself from the situation before you need to.

Coping strategies, understanding PMDD, and building a good relationship during the follicular phase aren't going to stop you from getting angry, but they reduce the risk of you raging and making associated poor decisions. The key is finding ways to increase your coping capacity during the luteal phase.

You, just like your partner, are susceptible to blaming other people or things when angry; remember that PMDD has a lot to answer for, but any relationship is more than just PMDD. You can't blame *everything* on PMDD (though it can account for an *awful lot*).

Where does PMDD end and your partner's personality begin? This is something that can only be learned with time, as each of you experiences the ups and downs that come with such a complex condition.

Compassion through communication.

We established earlier that your partner may not see any need to change during the luteal phase when they are angry, *there is a reduction in intention*, because of they feel a victim. Why should they change when *you* are responsible for those bad feelings? Change takes energy; it demands fuel; it needs *motivation*. There is likely little motivation to change during the luteal phase, as your partner may feel that their behaviour is fully justified.

If the motivation is not going to come from the person experiencing PMDD, then it might have to come from you. You must be convinced that you and your partner deserve a better life and be determined to try to achieve it. It is important to see your partner not as an enemy or opponent but as an ally —someone who is also working with you against a common enemy— PMDD. PMDD is the enemy that betrays both of you by mistreating you in different ways.

You can help your partner understand the effect that the rage has on both of you and your relationship by communicating this sympathetically and clearly during the follicular phase. There needs to be accountability to gain progress with PMDD. However, there may also be a need to communicate the extent of the harm that may be occurring during the luteal phase. If you are reaching the point where you are struggling to cope, tell your partner, *"I love you, but I am struggling to cope, I need to get some space to rebuild."* You may have to accept that such a statement might be interpreted negatively by your partner or that you are abandoning her, but it is crucial for *both of you* that you take the appropriate action for you to cope.

In the follicular phase, your emotional demeanour in communicating with your partner is important when discussing emotionally charged issues such as anger. It is probably more important than the words you use. Underpinned by genuine compassion, in your own words, it might go something like this:
"Neither of us is being the partner we want to be, I know that I'm not, and I'm fairly sure that in your heart you don't like the way we react to each other. If we go on like this, we will begin to hate ourselves. We have to try to become more understanding, sympathetic, and valuing of one another, for both of our sakes."

The most compassionate thing for you to do for your relationship is to be determined that there is a way you can be treated with the value and respect you deserve. Your relationship likely depends on it. It is in both your interests that the rage is managed to a level to keep the relationship from imploding. You are most humane when you model compassion and encourage your partner to do the same.

Why might the PMDD rage, anger, and dysphoria seem to be directed towards you?

Why do others not experience it in the same way?

How can your partner 'flip a switch' and behave differently to other people? Why is the majority of the rage directed at you and not others? This is often used by some partners to suggest that the dysphoria is "put on" or "can be controlled." I would strongly argue that this is not the case, but that there may be other reasons why the PMDD is targeted at specific individuals.

Ultimately, no one can really say with total authority why PMDD dysphoria might seem to be directed at you. The reasons are likely to be complex and a different dynamic is likely to exist in each relationship. Here are some thoughts ...

1. Reflect on your own behaviour.

It is possible that you might inadvertently make things worse. Reflect on your behaviour. Being patient, caring, empathetic, and treating your partner with respect is definitely going to help. There is so much value in considering and improving your own actions. However, remember that PMDD is not primarily caused by your behaviour so don't fall into the trap of blaming all your partner's dysphoria on yourself. PMDD, as far as we know, is an abnormal response to fluctuations in sex hormones. No matter how impeccable and agreeable your behaviour is, the dysphoria will still be there. Of course, when your behaviour is destructive, it worsens those symptoms, but consistent, immaculate behaviour doesn't alleviate them either. PMDD is not your fault, it's not her fault, it is just what it is: PMDD.

2. Your location.

You are probably more likely to experience it than other people because you are closest to it. You spend a lot of time with your partner. You have functional decisions to make together; you both have to figure out what to eat, where to go, and who does what. These decisions can present opportunities for points of conflict when the luteal phase hits.

3. "Masking"

Perhaps it is directed to you and not others for a different reason. Perhaps it is linked to the same reason kids misbehave for their parents, but wouldn't dare do it for an auntie, uncle, teacher or babysitter.

It's called masking. Masking is a facade; it's an illusion. It is to behave in a way that disguises true emotions or actions to fit in with those around them. It is normally done because a person wants to receive acceptance, and they might disguise characteristics like anger, jealousy, or rage – emotions that would not be considered socially acceptable.

Imagine you are in a job interview with complete strangers; both parties are going to be masking. You and the interviewer will be trying to keep great composure and convey a selected part of your personality.

You might be crumbling with nerves inside, but you mask those feelings to the best of your ability. It's exhausting! Partly, this is done out of protection; after all, you don't know how a stranger might react if you suddenly break down in tears or share a joke you think is really funny. You probably wouldn't get the job, and you would be upset if they reacted negatively.

When you meet someone for the first time, you don't share your full sense of humour or your darkest secrets. A relationship is built on progressively deepening trust and emotional risk. The less you know someone, the more likely you are to subconsciously be less intimate and more careful in your behaviour.

Masking like this takes great energy and only lasts for so long. Once unmasked, all those emotions are still there and still need to be processed.

(This happens in autism too; the symptoms are there but are 'masked' in public). Once the person is in a comfortable environment, the floodgates open and the true feelings spill out, sometimes generating a meltdown.

Your partner's fluctuating behaviour between you and other people isn't an indicator that your partner can stop it or switch her feelings on and off. It's more of an indicator that your partner can *temporarily redirect or hide it*. In a weird way, it's a compliment; it is saying, "I can be myself with you."

The deeper the relationship, the more comfortable with the person you become. It seems that close romantic partners or very close friends or family seem to occupy a special part of the brain. Think of the laughs you can have with close friends and people who really know you. Your partner trusts you and feels comfortable with you. You have seen her at her best and at her worst.

Perhaps paradoxically, the negativity of PMDD can be directed at you because she can subconsciously take off the mask she wears to the world.

4. PMDD needs reasons

Perhaps you have become a scapegoat for the awful PMDD dysphoria. We all naturally look for reasons to make sense of things that happen to us. Finding a reason for something helps make that experience more digestible in our minds.

It is recognised that there is self-serving bias occurring in all of us, and this can be very subconscious. Many of us will take credit for ourselves if things go well in life, but we may blame it on something else when things go bad. It may be that PMDD exacerbates and exaggerates this thought process.

For example, imagine taking a driver's test. If you pass the test, then you will likely make it an internal reason: I studied hard, I'm a naturally good driver. But if you fail the same test, suddenly there is an external reason— the weather was bad, it wasn't the car I usually drive, I didn't get enough sleep.

Blaming circumstances is one thing, but when things don't go well during PMDD and close partners are blamed, it can be harmful and severely damage relationships, families, and careers. When those with PMDD blame themselves, it can be equally destructive. Getting out of the 'blame game' of PMDD is liberating. PMDD might focus its attention on the behaviour of others to validate the desperately awful feelings of irritability or anger.

5. Depth of relationship

In any relationship, your partner already has a list of the things you do that they don't like. This is completely normal, but these differences don't normally really impair the relationship. PMDD hunts out those flaws in you or the relationship and feeds on them, inflating them until they become suffocating. The more intimate the relationship, the more evidence PMDD has to work with. Your relationship problems, character flaws, mistakes, or even existence can become targets for PMDD dysphoria.

Your partner's other, more superficial relationships with colleagues and acquaintances simply don't have the same depth or complexity as your own relationship, so there is scant material for the dysphoria to capitalise on. This means you may receive different treatment than other people.

"My partner tells it very clearly - during PMDD, she WANTS ME TO HATE HER, and a lot of her behaviour is directed towards creating this. In a way, the shame cycle brings one of the only forms of relief - if she makes me punish her or hate her, she feels that she deserved it, and that gives some kind of relief."

A partner, PMDD partner support Facebook page

6. A desperate plea for understanding.

There is something isolating about feeling anger and pain. When we experience it, we want people to understand it and know what we are going through.

Perhaps the rage, anger, and dysphoria are directed at you as a deep-seated subconscious method of trying to communicate the pain that is being felt by your partner. You are the one she loves the most and wants you to understand her the most.

The things you find joy in may become targets or triggers to your partner. Of course, making someone feel just as awful doesn't really help the situation; it just adds pain to an already painful situation.

Meltdowns

A cycle within a cycle.

Coping with PMDD when it is all kicking off

What people often want to know is how to react when their partner is having an acute episode. The luteal phase is a time when it can be very dark for the person experiencing it. It can also be incredibly lonely; no one can suffer it in her stead. The accumulation of intense symptoms can produce acute episodes of distress, creating extreme behaviour and emotions. The risk of harm is highest at this point, and it's a "PMDD meltdown." It is the acute moment of immediate stress when the dark clouds of PMDD produce enough friction to produce a sudden explosion and intense behaviour. It is the thunder and lightning of PMDD.

Understanding how to react can be really helpful in trying to calm the situation. It's the chapter I imagine most people flicking through the book will want to read first, as we are naturally drawn to the most urgent and important messages; however, if you really want to learn about how to reduce the risk or even prevent moments like these, then the preceding chapters on planning and relationship building are the best way to go. Planning, preparation, and patience! This chapter is more about "crisis handling," when things are acutely distressing. We will look at the anatomy of a meltdown, and then later we look a bit further into strategies to reduce conflict that might be associated with the meltdown.

No matter how well you prepare and no matter what lengths you will go to to provide the most harmonious situation for your partner, you will most likely find yourself in the "meltdown" situation from time to time (or more often!).

What is a PMDD meltdown?

Meltdowns are defined mental health events that can be predicted, analysed and even managed (to a degree). Meltdowns are an intense response to overwhelming situations and involve the person temporarily losing some amount of behavioural control. It is very common in those who have autism spectrum disorders, who, just like people with PMDD, can become overwhelmed in normal everyday situations. The meltdown occurs when the mind can't process or handle the intensity or complexity of the situation and, if we were to categorise, tends to be either explosive or catatonic.

A "**catatonic meltdown**" (shut down) is like using a PC, and Windows just decides to stop working; the screen freezes, the computer becomes unresponsive, and it tries to reset. What you might see in your partner during this time is a shut-down in communication, e.g. a loss of talking, reduced eye contact, defensive body language, making herself smaller (curling up), physically trying to remove herself from the situation, pulling a blanket over her head, etc. Although not as dramatic as an explosive meltdown, it is still a distressing episode.

An "**explosive meltdown**" This meltdown feels more dramatic-it's threatening and distressing, and it feels more out of control. It is noisy and unpredictable, and there often is a tidal wave of both non-verbal and verbal communication. Verbal communication presents as shouting, screaming, crying and threatening. Non-verbal communication may be physically hitting, lashing out, breaking objects or slamming doors.

Meltdowns are the body's way of coping with a situation it can't cope with. They act in many situations as a "reset" button. One might speculate that the evolutionary purpose of a meltdown is to change the dynamic of a situation quickly by more autonomic erratic, exaggerated behaviour so it becomes manageable. A meltdown feels primal. It is in the best interests of someone who is experiencing an intense experience (which they can't cope with) that their situation is changed quickly, even if it temporarily heightens the distress and emotions. The extreme behaviours of a meltdown usually manifest after the person has tried all available routes to cope with or avoid the situation and it doesn't work. The mind has no option but to press the "red" button that produces such dynamic and catastrophic behaviour, which means the situation *has* to change.

Safety Briefing: Emergency Crisis Situations

Firstly, a safety briefing. If during a meltdown the psychiatric symptoms that accompany PMDD descend to levels that are harmful, then you may need to consider the safety of those present, including your partner. Whilst I hope you never have to face these types of situations, the severity of PMDD is such that mental health can take a catastrophic nosedive. We are talking about the physical results of a mental health crisis: self-harm, suicide or other very self-destructive or dangerous behaviours, including violence. It is important to consider how you might respond, should the situation arise, or reflect on how you have handled previous situations.

The ideal is that during an acute mental health crisis (I know I am repeating myself) you and your partner have a support plan in place. It should be written together in the follicular phase, and it should state **what you should do** as a partner in each situation. It is an opportunity to plan when you both are cool headed and there is space to think. That agreement removes some of the uncertainty or self-doubt about what is appropriate and it gives you the confidence to make appropriate interventions. Care planning also helps create boundaries. Topics may cover self-harm, violence, and suicide. Be as specific and detailed as possible. If your partner won't write one, write one for yourself, as your capacity to make good decisions may be impaired in the heat of the moment.

While a person's self-autonomy and self-determination are generally untouchable, there are some exceptions where safety is concerned. It might feel uncomfortable to call on professionals against your partner's wishes, perhaps it will feel like a breach of trust, **but the things that matter most should never be at the mercy of the things that matter least**. Safety first—your partner's safety and your own safety.

If someone was having a heart attack, you wouldn't wait for permission to call an ambulance, right? If you discovered someone lying unconscious on the street, would you pull up a chair and wait for them to regain consciousness so you can chat about whether they want an ambulance or not? In both cases, the sufferer's capacity to respond to the situation themselves has diminished to the point that they are in danger.

You will need to tread very carefully if you need to contact a professional on your partner's behalf, and only do it if it is right to do so. If you are unsure, and you find yourself sitting on a fence, it is better to err on the side of safety. Contact the professionals. The situations requiring you to contact professionals are where you, family members or your partner are at risk of harm:

- Your partner has harmed themselves and needs medical attention.
- You feel they might act on suicidal feelings.
- They are putting themselves or someone else at immediate, serious risk of harm (someone else includes you).

During an acute PMDD episode/meltdown, ask yourself, "Are they safe?"

If they are not safe by themselves, stay with them or at a distance where you may be able to observe their safety and help them call for an ambulance. If they won't call for an ambulance and they need it, call it for them. Many places in the UK have what are called "crisis teams" for acute mental health problems that provide service in these types of situations. During an acute PMDD meltdown, your partner may not want you anywhere around, which makes it difficult to ensure their safety. Ideally, prior to the episode, an agreement is reached between partner and sufferer that recognises the need to ensure safety. If you are in a separate place and you are concerned for their safety, call for help.

If they are safe by themselves for a while, then there are other services that can be accessed, e.g. an emergency appointment with the family doctor, and mental health telephone services. In the UK, we have the phone number "111," which is for non-emergency situations. It would be wise to remove anything around the person that could be used for harm.
There are some good resources online for dealing with someone who is suicidal, should you need them.[39]

---

[39] Supporting someone with suicidal feeling- Mind: https://www.mind.org.uk/information-support/helping-someone-else/supporting-someone-who-feels-suicidal/about-suicidal-feelings/

If you feel in immediate danger, or you have already been harmed, call the police. If other people, e.g. children or relatives, are in immediate danger, call the police. Don't mess around. Don't overthink it. If people are in danger, including yourself, you have a duty to everyone, including your partner, to call the police. Although you will probably worry about getting your partner in trouble, it is for her own protection as well as your for own. You are protecting her and yourself from the extreme mental health symptoms that can come from PMDD. It is important to make it clear to your partner that there are lines that, if crossed, you will take appropriate action, but do this in the right way and at the right time. Perhaps it will act as a prompt for your partner to recognise how extreme the condition has become if external organisations are becoming involved.

In the next section, we look in detail at the 'meltdown' anatomy. There was a lot of focus during the COVID global pandemic on "flattening the curve" (at least in the UK), which meant that lockdown measures would prevent an extremely high spike in infection rates. The virus was going to spread no matter what in the end, but *flattening the curve* was all about trying to delay or diminish the peak. To flatten the curve in PMDD is to starve it of fuel or energy. Like the virus – it is going to come into her life regardless, but I want to run through some ideas about reducing the harm and intensity of those acute PMDD moments.

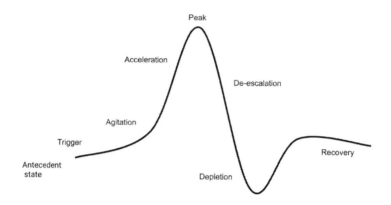

The Anatomy of a PMDD Meltdown

Meltdowns have a predictable cycle, and once you reflect on previous experiences, you will notice the pattern. Knowledge of how the meltdown runs is crucial, so you can adjust your own behaviour to each stage.

The antecedent stage

This is the pre-existing state that your partner is in prior to any meltdown.

What is your partner's current mood or disposition?

Is it heightened? Is there a stressful social event coming up? Work deadline? Listen to what your partner is saying—she may hopefully be telling you directly how she feels, but if she isn't, she will be telling you through her behaviour, body language, demeanour, or other activities. Intervention at this stage should focus on reducing the risk of your partner reaching the meltdown stage through de-escalation.

If you have a good idea of your partner's antecedent stage, then you will be able to help redirect or remove potential triggers, or you will at least have some sort of warning that a crescendo is imminent. A good method can be energy accounting- which is discussed later in the book.

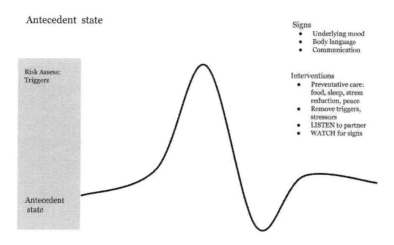

Antecedent state

Signs
- Underlying mood
- Body language
- Communication

Risk Assess:
Triggers

Interventions
- Preventative care: food, sleep, stress reduction, peace
- Remove triggers, stressors
- LISTEN to partner
- WATCH for signs

Antecedent state

It's hard to live with someone and not know what triggers them or what their vulnerabilities are. Remember, on balance, PMDD "inflates and exaggerates" more than it "creates." The vast majority of the existing problems, paranoias, self-doubts, and other vulnerabilities would still be there even without PMDD, but at a much-reduced level. If you fancy a bit of happy reading on a Friday night (outside the luteal phase), perhaps ask your partner to list all her triggers. While I am half-joking about doing this, it isn't a bad idea if your partner is willing, to engage and make a few notes, as the more you know and understand about the triggers, the better you are able to anticipate and negate potential triggers and, in turn, meltdowns. Obviously, if you do decide to ask your partner to list all the potential triggers, you may naturally find a lot of your own behaviour on that list, and so you must be cool-headed enough to *just listen without comment.* Your partner may list some triggers that seem incredulous or ridiculous to you - they may actually be incredulous or ridiculous. It doesn't matter. She is not you, and you are not her. In those moments, the triggers are very real. If this truly is a listening exercise, then the goal is to know what the triggers are, not analysing the validity of the triggers. Ultimately, if they are important to her, then it's worth knowing about them and taking them into account regardless of whether you think they are silly. Prevention at the antecedent stage is about anticipation and reading the situation.

If you can see the descent in mood and can anticipate a meltdown is going to occur, remove as many of the triggers as you can. Will your presence help the situation? Are you the trigger? Sometimes it can be hard to walk away from a situation when you know your partner is distressed. If you leave, will you be later accused of walking away from or abandoning your partner? Are you worried about what she may do if she is alone and vulnerable? Conversely, will your presence make things worse? Does she want you there? Do you want to be near her because you can't bear the thought of someone you love suffering alone? Ask her. What is in your predetermined care plan? Meltdown risk reduction occurs when your partner feels more in control of the situation.

"What can I do to help you right now?"

"I want to help you, but I am not sure how. Can you tell me?"

"Do you want me to stay, or would you like some time and space?"

Regardless of where you are geographically— next to her or in another room— there are things you can do to help reduce the risk of a meltdown. What stressors can I remove from her situation? Can I reschedule that visit or delay that deadline? What flexibility is there that I can adjust? It is around this time that providing a calming environment, or other comforts that soothe— food, candles or a bath—*might* help.

PMDD diminishes the sufferer's sense of self-autonomy. It must be scary to suddenly feel that you no longer have the same control over your emotions and wellbeing.

This loss of self-determination and control is heightened in the acute phase. Many people with PMDD have remarked that sometimes their memory is cloudy of what happened when they had a PMDD meltdown or even that they can't remember. It is true that they may genuinely not remember some of the things that have been said. One of the ways you can help keep the antecedent state low is to *restore that sense of control.*

Listening to your partner's concerns, affirming behaviours, not over-questioning, giving her space where she wants it, not coercing her to attend functions and respecting her self-autonomy are all things that keep the antecedent state low. Also avoid making demands or giving commands! Be agile to a changing situation. Proactive actions like promoting rest, preparing food, and keeping the environment calm may pay dividends in avoiding a major meltdown.

Remember that even with or without your interventions, a meltdown may occur, and you shouldn't feel guilty if it happens despite your best efforts. You have not failed if your partner has a meltdown; her mental state is not a direct consequence of your every action! Go easy on yourself and do not blame yourself. It's not her fault, and it's not your fault. PMDD is just "there"—it exists without blame or permission.

Trigger, agitation and acceleration

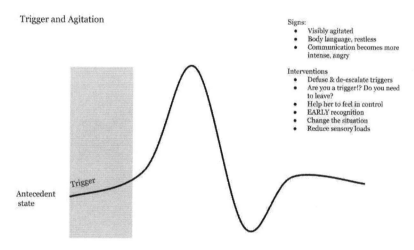

Trigger and Agitation

Signs:
- Visibly agitated
- Body language, restless
- Communication becomes more intense, angry

Interventions
- Defuse & de-escalate triggers
- Are you a trigger!? Do you need to leave?
- Help her to feel in control
- EARLY recognition
- Change the situation
- Reduce sensory loads

Trigger

Antecedent state

Once the trigger has been pulled, the manageable becomes unmanageable, and there seems to be a self-reinforcing downward spiral. It's like watching a car crash. You know what is happening, you know what will happen, and you anticipate the damage. You will see the acceleration of symptoms, the distress becoming more intense, and the behaviour becoming more erratic and unpredictable. If your partner can leave the situation or remove the trigger, then this is probably *the last opportunity to avoid the full meltdown*. The further along the cycle, the more the emotional and subconscious autonomic systems seem to control your partner's behaviour. It is like something very primal kicks in. Calming techniques are less likely to work, and it is also not a time to make requests, ask lots of questions, or request your partner do something. She is struggling to cope with the situation, and adding more responsibility or requests serves only to overload her and becomes a catalyst for escalation.

Around this time, PMDD will be looking for a reason for the meltdown. If a clear reason can't be found, then PMDD will create one. Baiting is a good way for PMDD to try and legitimise anger. Baiting is when your partner deliberately annoys or provokes you for a reaction. Once your partner gets a reaction from you, then *you* become the cause of the argument. It's not the unpleasant experience she is going through or the feelings of dysphoria; it's you (or at least that's how they feel in that moment). It may be that you are described as the problem in the relationship and that she would be better off without you.

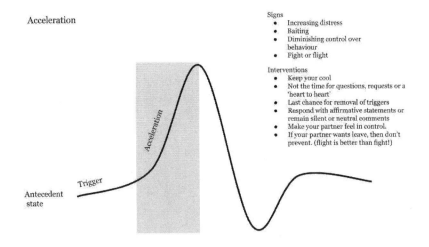

146

It is an attempt to flip the situation, your partner blames you, who are more likely to be innocent.

Your partner may become angrier by your responses, and her provoking becomes justified because your angry responses prove that it was "*you who started it*" and she is simply defending herself. By blaming you for the argument, attention is diverted from her own behaviour. You are often left confused and feeling manipulated.

The key to avoiding reinforcing this behaviour is to not give in and to stand your ground through the baiting process. By this, I mean that you do not become antagonistic, argue, or offensively react to the baiting, but rather you stand firm in who you are and are able to calmly deflect anything that is thrown at you. You dig in and either take the strain or leave the situation and wait for clarity of mind. The latter is probably the better of the two options. If you can't remove yourself from the situation, like soldiers of Gondor, "Whatever comes through those doors, stand your ground."

This is the moment when you find a space inside you, an internal peace, a purpose that PMDD cannot infiltrate. For some people, this may be a religious centre or a spiritual strength; for others, it may be the firm logic that this behaviour is not who your partner is and that it is PMDD talking. This is why every partner of someone with PMDD says that the most important and profound advice that can be given is simply, "Separate the person from the condition."

After some years of practice, it never got to the point where the rage of PMDD didn't hurt me in some way. However, the internal peace grew, and it felt like I could deflect most of the arrows that were fired, and their penetration was lessened. It wasn't a case of having thicker skin; I am still a sensitive soul.[40] It was more that I was like Neo in the Matrix, suddenly seeing everything for what it really was. This meant that I couldn't necessarily be hurt in the same way. I could slow down the bullets and dodge them. Understanding PMDD is a superpower.

---

[40] I cried watching The Notebook.

Peak

Peak is the most uncomfortable and distressing part of the meltdown. You are both at the "peak," and you are both standing on the line between giving up and seeing how much more you can take. It is the extremes of life. This is primal survival mode, and your partner may do whatever is needed to get through the next few minutes or hours. Your partner may *feel* out of control and may *act* out of control. There may be helpings of verbal abuse. No vulnerability or insecurity you have

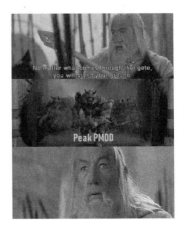

is off limits. You can't really do much once the peak is on except try to keep things safe, including yourself. If you are in danger, you must remove yourself from the situation. If others are in danger, then you should remove them from the situation. If your partner is a danger to herself, then you may need to contact the local mental health crisis team. At the height of the peak, you can't talk or reason, and it is certainly not the time to solve problems. Luckily, the peak can only be sustained for so long because it is physically demanding on the body's resources, and the intensity will naturally reduce after an uncomfortable period of time.

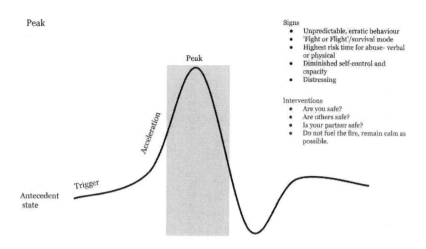

My wife would find it most difficult to talk about the times when PMDD was at its worst. Understandably, sufferers feel responsible for the things they do and say and the guilt is immense. I feel many underestimate how much of someone's behaviour can be accounted for by PMDD. Even those who have PMDD, may not appreciate how severe it can be. In a relationship, you develop a sense of who someone is—their character, and their outlook—and that should be markedly different from what you see during PMDD in a healthy relationship.

I was lucky in the sense that my wife is a truly lovely person, and so the gulf between PMDD and normality was more demarcated. In my 17 years of experience with my wife, I know who she is, and I do not hold her responsible for those acute episodes. They did not represent who she is or the principles she lives by. Additionally, meltdowns would not, with the odd exception, occur at times other than the luteal phase of PMDD. Presumably, if my theory that PMDD was responsible for the majority of the meltdowns and aberrant behaviour was correct, then presumably these behaviours would vanish after a complete hysterectomy and oophorectomy. If it stayed after the surgery, then this behaviour was just part of my wife and my life. My position was vindicated following surgery; these acute meltdowns ceased with time, and the wife I had for half the month stayed for the rest of the month. There are still bumps in the road after the surgery as her body continues to adjust to a surgical menopause and taking HRT, but I would now consider her symptoms to be 95% reduced.

The view from "the peak." Your partner will express the most intense emotions at the peak. You hear the phrase "fight or flight" and that accurately describes what may happen during a meltdown: our partner's instinctual brain wiring switches the person into "survival mode" as a coping mechanism. It may be that your partner shuts down, withdraws, or tries to escape the situation. Alternatively, meltdowns may be catastrophic. The most intense emotions are displayed outwardly in a catastrophic meltdown—raising her voice, becoming more animated, and, in some cases escalating to shouting, swearing, etc. The extreme end of a catastrophic meltdown may be physical expressions of rage and might involve kicking, hitting, throwing objects, or damaging things. Your partner may end your relationship or exit the situation. It is the end of days; the world is falling apart. It is the desperation of someone caged, trapped, and left out of control by a vicious cycle that makes them feel there is no other way for them to cope with the situation.

It is important to note that once in this frame of mind, the person experiencing the meltdown has reduced capacity to process information, reason, and rationalise during the height of the meltdown due to the overwhelming symptoms.

It may seem obvious, but it follows that no problems are ever fixed during peak. Really, don't even attempt to try and fix things; don't try to talk things over. It is not the time to make requests or introduce changes. It only fuels the fire as any action you perform may be interpreted as a negative gesture, and "anything you do say may be used as evidence against you." Trying to solve problems at their peak is like trying to build a house back up when it is burning. If you want to stop the fire, you starve it of oxygen and give it time. If you want to feed the fire, you add fuel to the flames.

During the peak, avoid threats or provocative moves. This only fuels the meltdown further. Think: Has this approach ever helped the situation before? As you stand immovable, with a calm sense of security about what PMDD looks like, you can detach your emotions and those of your partner.

If I were to summarise how to deal with a meltdown during the peak, I would say the following mnemonic is useful as a reference: the "SCALED" approach to a PMDD meltdown:

Safe	Ensure that everyone is safe, including you, your partner, and family members.
Calm[41]	Calm the situation and try to keep calm yourself.
Affirmation	Affirm your support and care
Listen	Listen to concerns and continue to affirm
Environment	Make the environment more conducive for recovery
Distinguish	Distinguish between PMDD and normal healthy behaviour; separate the person.

Or if you would like a shorter one...

PMDD: **P**revent, **M**anage, **D**e-escalate, **D**ebrief![42]

---

[41] Calming down starts with you and finishes with them (hopefully!)
[42] Debrief during the follicular phase

De-escalation and Post-crisis Depletion

Allow rest and recovery. A meltdown is such an intense emotional, mental, and physiological cataclysmic eruption that it cannot be sustained for a long time. The body is regulating its response, and it needs rest, so it is perfectly normal to feel absolutely shattered after. Like someone who has just run a marathon, your partner may feel drained, tired, and vulnerable. The de-escalation stage is awash with a strange grief, littered with dark thoughts and hopelessness. Your partner's self-control and reflective processes are gradually returning. This may be minutes, but it is more likely to be hours or the rest of the day as the melancholy weariness of PMDD rests heavy on the shoulders of its subject.

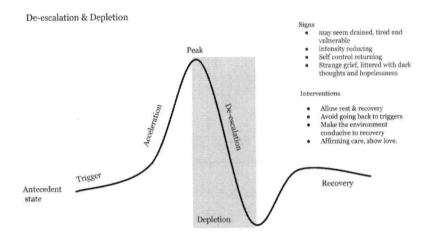

De-escalation & Depletion

Peak

Signs
- may seem drained, tired and vulnerable
- Intensity reducing
- Self control returning
- Strange grief, littered with dark thoughts and hopelessness

Interventions
- Allow rest & recovery
- Avoid going back to triggers
- Make the environment conducive to recovery
- Affirming care, show love.

Acceleration

De-escalation

Trigger

Antecedent state

Recovery

Depletion

Avoid going back to triggers unless you want to do it all again. There is a time to talk about things, but likely not when your partner is tired, vulnerable, or grieving. Instead of picking apart the last few hours, reset your mind and offer support and love. Affirmation during the most vulnerable times is an emotional deposit that pays interest. You might feel angry, upset, and persecuted, and you will have to communicate those feelings to her at the right time and in the right way, but perhaps another time; for now, extending compassion or giving her space is the best option. It takes time to recover and rebuild.

Make the environment conducive to recovery. Where possible, try to create a quiet, safe space. If in public, ask people to move along, find a private place, turn off loud music and avoid anything that may distract your partner from recovering. Whatever you can think of to reduce the overload, try it.

Consider your own meltdown

Consider now the journey your partner has gone through an absolute rollercoaster. I have written this from the point of view of someone who is an objective bystander, neutrally observing the sequence of events from space. The truth is she wasn't alone on this cycle—you went through it too. You experienced some of the same feelings as she did, probably in the same order and at the same time.

Consider how tied your emotions are to hers. You are sitting side by side on the rollercoaster, and you can't expect to feel apathetic when you are so emotionally tied to

> Since the moods are so all-consuming (as my gf describes them), it feels almost like they're trying to consume you with them too. Projection is pretty common in a PMDD episode, and if they're projecting their own feelings of depression and rage onto us then we are going to feel that way too.
>
> PMDD Partner, PMDD forum

someone. Their hurt is yours, and your hurt is theirs. When they get angry, you probably get angry too. When they feel sad, you feel sad. If you reciprocate her feelings, then you risk reinforcing her feelings and that may cause exacerbation of the dysphoric feelings.

The big difference between her experience and what you experience is the amount of control you have and the ability to detach from the narrative. Obviously, the amount of control over our own emotions varies between individuals, but generally, partners who are not experiencing PMDD should be able to exert more self-control, and so it behoves us as partners to take that self-control and maximise it.

To flatten the curve in PMDD is to starve it of fuel or energy. Engaging in the argument, taking the bait, and becoming angrier yourself are all things that will fuel the meltdown. Try to remain in control of your own feelings and recognise that a lot of what is said during PMDD is not truly representative of how she feels. During PMDD, there could even be an element of paranoia or even conspiracy; things that are demonstrably false suddenly become true. Being repeatedly exposed to misinformation of this nature starts to make you question your own sense of truth and reality. It is also true that there could be very hurtful things said; early on in our relationship, it was shattering to my confidence. I was just trying to be the best husband I could be, and yet I felt like the worst human. It felt like it didn't matter how central I made the welfare of my wife, it would not be good enough, and I felt hated for my failure and hated myself.

When you separate the person from the condition, it empowers you to deal in a more objective way and recognise what is happening. Just like a cough is a symptom of a cold, the rage and paranoia can be transient symptoms of PMDD. Let the symptoms wash over you; don't inhale them as they are toxic. Try not to take them personally; they don't define you.

Conflict Management

When something like that happens in my marriage, I slow down, take a breath, and try to acknowledge myself to myself. I acknowledge what my intentions are, I acknowledge what I have invested in the relationship, and I acknowledge the limitations I am feeling. I tell myself "Hey man, I know you're just trying your best". This helps me feel a lot less high stakes in the moment. Sometimes it helps me think of a creative or empathetic way to reengage with my wife. Other times, it helps me advocate for myself needing my own space to get okay and think. Often times both my wife and I are better at noticing what's going on after a few minutes of space. And even if she's still frustrated or aggravated, I'm in a much better headspace and know what I can capacitate that given night.

Partner, PMDD forum.

There is repeated debate between partners in support groups about how to deal with the conflict that can arise with PMDD. How do you deal with the conflict in PMDD? It is well recognised that accusations and agitated arguments arise frequently in the luteal phase.

Do you fight back?

If you feel you are right, you should stick to your guns, right?

Should you just roll over and let it "all go"?

By doing nothing in that moment, are you enabling? Are you reinforcing "bad" behaviour?

Are there other approaches you can take?

Conflict Soup

As much as I have emphasised the preference to discuss difficult things during the follicular phase rather than the luteal phase, there are going to be times when delaying a disagreement or decision isn't possible, after all you probably live together and some decisions can't wait until the next stage of the menstrual cycle. We can't always prevent, avoid or circumvent having conflict in a relationship, sometimes we just have *to get through it*. Disagreements are natural parts of relationships and fighting right is a skill!

Conflicts are like a weird soup, full of emotional ingredients that get mixed up in one hell of a hot sticky confusing mess. But it doesn't always have to be like that. Every disagreement has consistent components and can be broken down. Once you dissect a disagreement or argument, it becomes easier to cope with and easier to resolve. In short, you can reverse engineer an argument.

For most disagreements there are four main ingredients:
- Observations
- Thoughts
- Emotions
- Wants

These ingredients in the soup are all floating around in the liquid of 'previous experiences,' such as past traumas and relationships. Our previous experiences frame our future responses.

This model called the Experience Cube[43] has almost universal application. In using this model, it doesn't matter if your partner has PMDD or not, PMDD just seems to just turn up the heat and makes the conflict soup

---

[43] By Gervase R. Bushe https://coachingleaders.co.uk/the-experience-cube-explained-in-a-page/

harder to work with! Let's look at each ingredient and how it contributes to the flavour of the disagreement.

At the base of most disagreements is an **unmet need or a want**, and finding *what that need is* can be difficult as we often express ourselves in confusing ways. Even if you feel the unmet need is *only* PMDD, it rarely is, it is more likely there is a vulnerability, a need or a want that PMDD is exacerbating.

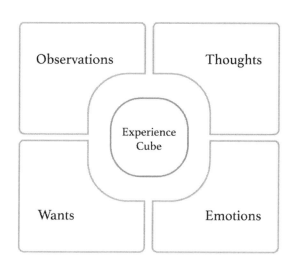

The Experience Cube is a useful model to help pick-apart what is happening in conflict.

There are four interconnected elements:

1. Observations: These are the tangible things we perceive through our senses—what we see, hear, touch, taste, and smell. *Observations are the raw material* and we use them to build the rest of our experience.

2. Thoughts: Our beliefs, internal dialogue, and interpretations fall into this category. *Thoughts shape how we perceive an experience* and shape our emotions and are often prompted by what we observe.

3. Emotions: Feelings arise from our thoughts and observations. They colour our experience and significantly impact our behaviour.

4. Wants: These represent our desires, goals, and intentions. What do we hope to achieve? What outcomes do we seek?

	Observations	Thoughts	Feelings	Wants
Jude	Jude notices that Aaron seems distant and less affectionate during her PMDD phase	Jude thinks, "Aaron doesn't care about me anymore. He's pulling away."	Jude feels hurt, abandoned, and anxious	Jude wants reassurance, understanding, and emotional support
Aaron	Aaron observes that Jude becomes irritable and sensitive	Aaron thinks, "Jude is always overreacting. Why can't she just relax?"	Aaron experiences frustration and annoyance	Aaron wants peace, harmony and avoiding conflict.

During conflicts people often confuse each other's thoughts, interpretations and observations of an event, forgetting that someone can have the same thing happen to them and feel completely different.

Conversations end up defensive and accusatory. **Facts and events can be the same, but our observations can be so different** - a bit like how my wife and I feel differently about roller coasters. They make Jude feel great and they make me feel sick! We might both come off that roller coaster, she might say, "That rollercoaster was amazing! whilst I firmly say, "That roller coaster was the worst!" Yet we sat together on the same roller coaster.

Each person is entitled to their own interpretation of an event, even if it is far removed from the facts of what happened. The difficulty comes when people present their experience as an irrefutable fact and enforce their interpretation as the only one. Anger only seems to increase the confidence people have in their own perceptions, making it more challenging to see another point of view.

During conflicts it is helpful to avoid language that sounds accusatory. **"I statements"** are a communication technique used to express your feelings and needs in a clear and assertive way, without attaching blame or accusing your partner. Here's a breakdown of their use:

- **Start with "I":** This personal pronoun immediately centres the statement on your experience.
- **Describe the situation:** Briefly explain the situation that led to your feelings.
- **Express your feelings:** Use clear and specific emotional words like "frustrated," "hurt," "excited," or "proud." Avoid accusatory terms like, "You made me feel..."
- **(Optional!) State the impact:** Briefly explain how the situation affected you.
- **(Optional!) State your needs:** If appropriate, express what you would like to see happen.

For example:

You-Statement: "You never listen to me when I talk about work!" (Focuses on blame and sounds and accusatory)

I-Statement: "I feel frustrated when I talk about my day at work and it feels like you're distracted. I would love to hear your thoughts about it." (Focuses on feelings and expresses a need)

Being able to help someone separate the event from blame, accusations, thoughts and feelings is *so* useful. It's moving from a mentality where one of you has to win and the other has to lose the argument, to one where there is mutual understanding. It's not about who is right, it's about what is right to resolve the situation. We must find the common ground to start back again and be able to separate out our interpretations. You will likely have more success in dealing with her **wants and needs** and address those rather than going back over the initial observation. Using the example given previously, Aaron will have more success in resolving the argument by addressing Jude's wants of reassurance and emotional support than trying to prove to her that she was distant and less affectionate. In this case, concentrating on her 'cold' behaviour rather than her want for reassurance could probably worsen the situation. That's why rather than asking "What's wrong?" it is better to ask, "What can I do to help you?".

The cascade of observations, thoughts, feelings and wants were what *we experienced*. If her experience is wildly different than yours, it doesn't invalidate our own experience, it just means there is a wide gulf between our interpretations of an event. You can't take ownership of her experience, it's hers. But you can make efforts to try and understand it and what *want* she wanted to communicate to you.

Paul in a support group wisely said
"Your feelings are yours, and they are based on your thoughts or interpretations of facts (what actually happened).
Keep the facts separate from the impact of the facts on you. She may have shouted, disappeared on your anniversary, or whatever - those are the facts. Why she did that and how you felt about that are your interpretation and experience. The benefit of that for you is that she can't deny the facts, and she can't deny your experience. The benefit for her is that she doesn't have to own your experience, either.
You can ask for a change in behaviour and she can refuse, but you've articulated why you want the behaviour change based on how it impacted you. It also gives her opportunity to share an alternative thought process."

A good example is that I found during PMDD my wife would often resent things that brought me joy. Whether it was surfing or spending time with friends. I couldn't work out why she would resent my feeling happy. If she loved me and wanted the best for me, then surely these fulfilling parts of my life wouldn't be points of conflict and resentment. It seemed a little vindictive.

Seven years after having surgery and PMDD is no longer in our lives the way it was, this subject came up in conversation. Jude told me she resented these hobbies and activities because they gave me the joy she felt she couldn't offer as a partner. My heart broke into a thousand pieces for her.

It was a perspective so oblique and bizarre to me, without her telling me I would never have worked it out.

By understanding each other's observations, thoughts, emotions, and wants, it can be possible to navigate PMDD-related disagreements with compassion and clarity.
We can give our relationships a fighting chance.

Attachment Styles

A useful model to use when discussing relationships and conflicts are *attachment styles*. For further reading on the subject, I recommend the PhD thesis by Dr Rose Alkattan[44] that looks at the experiences of partners of those with PMDD.

Attachment styles can be a useful lens to look at the way you and your partner interact. Like any theory or model, it has a limit to how much it can apply to an individual. The reality is we probably are a blend of the different styles or are just weighted more to one particular attachment style. Regardless, it's a useful exercise to view your relationships through. For those with PMDD, their attachment style may vary depending on where they are in the cycle.

The theory of attachment styles was developed by British psychologist John Bowlby. He proposed that young children have an innate need for emotional closeness and security, and they develop attachment bonds to their primary caregivers (usually their parents) as a way to meet these needs.

People seem to really like the theory, and it has been applied to understand not only romantic relationships but also parent-child relationships, friendships, and even therapeutic relationships. So now we are applying it to PMDD relationships.

There are four primary attachment styles:

Secure Attachment: People with secure attachment styles feel comfortable with emotional intimacy and independence. They tend to have positive views of themselves and their partners, and they can trust and rely on their partners while maintaining a healthy sense of individuality. If you are someone with a secure attachment style in a PMDD relationship, you may find it easier than others to demonstrate understanding and support

---

[44] Dr Rose Alkattan
https://digitalcommons.liberty.edu/cgi/viewcontent.cgi?article=5902&context=doctoral

when your partner experiences PMDD symptoms. You may have the capacity to offer more emotional stability and consistency during difficult times.

Securely attached partners can be a significant source of comfort and empathy for individuals with PMDD.

Anxious-Preoccupied Attachment: Individuals with this style may seek high levels of emotional closeness and need a lot of validation in their relationships. They may worry about their partner's commitment (which is easy to do in a PMDD relationship) and constantly seek reassurance. This attachment style can lead to relationship challenges when their needs aren't met.

It makes sense that if you have an anxious-preoccupied attachment style you may experience more heightened anxiety and insecurity than others when your partner is going through PMDD.

If you are this attachment style then you are probably a lot more prone to interpret PMDD symptoms as personal rejection, leading to more conflicts and misunderstandings. It is, therefore crucial to work on communication and self-calming/reassuring techniques during PMDD episodes.

Dismissive-Avoidant Attachment: Those with a dismissive-avoidant attachment style often emphasise self-sufficiency and independence. They may have difficulty relying on or opening up to their partners, appearing emotionally distant at times. They may be more prone to expecting others to be self-sufficient or independent too, even if they have PMDD. Vulnerability and intimacy can be challenging for people with this style.

You can imagine that if you have a dismissive-avoidant attachment style, you may struggle to provide emotional support during PMDD episodes. You might distance yourself from your partner, or perhaps adopt this style in the luteal phase. Dismissiveness could lead to viewing the emotional fluctuations as a burden. Open communication and understanding the cyclical nature of PMDD can help bridge the gap for these types of relationships.

Fearful-Avoidant Attachment (Disorganised Attachment): People with this style have a copious dashing of anxious and avoidant tendencies. They are confusing! They may both desire and fear emotional intimacy, leading to a push-pull dynamic in their relationships. Expect a hectic mix of ambivalence and fluctuating emotions. We all know that PMDD can trigger intense emotional responses, and if you are a fearful-avoidant partner, then the conflict of all the emotions can be overwhelming and you might feel that you just simply can't handle the situation. Ideally, if you are this style, therapy to address your own issues could be helpful.

Once you consider the approach you and your partner have to each other, you can start to mesh your attachment styles vs how you both manage conflict.

There are many recognised strategies and models for managing conflict. The Thomas Kilmann Model[45] is a thought exercise in how conflict can be resolved. It has two main components that seem to battle each other for priority when resolving conflicts. These two components are:

assertiveness and cooperation.

Assertiveness is all about what *you want,* and cooperation is what *they want.* Let's take a look at different approaches to the conflict within PMDD. I am not saying there is one particular approach that is the right approach; in different situations, you have to make a judgement call. It is a case of deciding which of the options you have is **best for the situation**. The following notes are more of a *prompt to think,* or an *invitation to reflect* on the approaches you take to conflict in the relationship.

---

[45] For a brief overview of the model the following Youtube video is useful. https://www.youtube.com/watch?v=PFIydyH2H8Y

We are going to look at the four aspects of conflict:

- Avoidance

- Accommodation

- Collaboration

- Competition

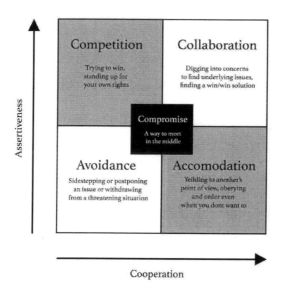

1. Avoidance

Avoidance mostly tries to ignore or sidestep the conflict, hoping it will resolve itself or dissipate. This is quite often a good technique in PMDD for an **acute** situation, as the most symptoms dissipate naturally through the cycle. Sometimes the point of an argument is something that just won't matter once the luteal phase is over.

It's not that you are avoiding it because it is easier or because you are being cowardly, it is a thoughtful, calculated approach that reduces conflict and limits the damage of PMDD to a relationship. Obviously in most situations avoiding dealing with problems like PMDD is just *not* sustainable in the long term and eventually things come to a head. But as a short-term strategy, avoiding (combined with healthy discussions when everyone feels better later on) can be an effective method. The cyclical nature of PMDD means that suddenly the problem of a few days ago is no longer a problem and a lot of heartache would be spared by avoiding dragging it up. It reminds me of the WORST advice given at weddings and bounced around social media: "Never go to sleep on an argument." Who came up with this? I find after sleep, the new morning brings a clarity to my mind and a bit more rationality. Sleep is the body's reset button.

As discussed earlier in the book, PMDD also magnifies existing problems, so it is worth making a mental note of some of the issues that are raised and seeing if they can be discussed at an appropriate time, especially if it is important to you. PMDD can't be side-stepped or ignored – but avoiding certain subjects during high tensions is an effective way to help reduce the damage that PMDD can cause.

One down side is that during acute PMDD situations your partner may recognise you are taking this technique, she may feel aggrieved at you trying to dodge issues that she feels are important at that moment. You may try to face this by using affirmative statements about how you recognise the points being raised are important, but they may be best discussed at another time (by which you may feel stretched, worn down and ready to say, "Enough is enough!").

2. Accommodation

"Giving in" to these demands seems wrong. It feels like defeat! Especially when you don't agree with them. I felt that accommodating some of the most unreasonable demands would have been an affront to my identity and my ability to preserve self-autonomy, so I would regularly resist. However, resisting was a sure way of being accused of being unsupportive or unloving and would feed into false narratives during PMDD or, at worst, could lead to a catastrophic meltdown.

The alternative of just doing everything she wanted and almost giving up my self-identity and self-government during the luteal phase also seemed soul-destroying and unachievable. The level of perfection required in every task and aspect of life felt insurmountable. Even Gandhi would struggle. If you accommodate everything your partner wants and everything revolves around her during PMDD, is that really the way to live a life? Are you enabling or reinforcing behaviour?

Self-determination is a fundamental precept of life. I would hear in my mind the quote my grandfather recited to me once: "Anyone who lives their life entirely the way someone else wants them to live is either pathetic or a politician." Yet again, with PMDD, it feels like you are stuck between a rock and a hard place with two equally damaging alternatives.

The solution is often found in the delicate nuance of compromise. Can you make *reasonable accommodations*? If the trigger is the method you use to load the dishwasher, is it really too much to ask to just let this one go? Is it really the hill you want to die upon? However, if your partner wants you to sever ties with friends who are important to you, perhaps this is a different type of accommodation that is not so appropriate.

Deciding not to accommodate your PMDD partner's wishes is a "withdrawal" from that bank account and should be carefully thought out. Sometimes providing clear boundaries may seem like a withdrawal to the relationship in the short term, but in the long term it is a deposit in that bank account. Don't act out of stubbornness; act out of careful consideration. There are times when accommodating smaller issues is worth doing. Especially in an escalating situation where there is a high risk of meltdown.

Giving in doesn't mean you are giving up.

It means that you can rationally decide what is most important. I guess it is a form of "choosing your battles."

There is a balance to be struck. You must preserve some self-autonomy but also limit the damage of PMDD. Therefore, when you accommodate her requests, it is a conscious act of self-determination and identity. You are making your own choices, even if it is occasionally to do something you think isn't a good idea!

3. Compromising and Collaboration

The art of "compromise" involves finding an acceptable resolution that will partly, but not entirely, satisfy the concerns of all parties involved. A compromised solution may be difficult to find in the midst of the luteal phase.

Finding a solution is possible during the luteal phase, but the symptoms can be so intense during PMDD that your partner might lack the capacity to engage. Remember, as discussed previously, during PMDD, your partner might have a diminished concept of others' feelings and wants. Finding a good compromise is a delicate process that requires good communication and a willingness to understand from both parties. If that can be present during PMDD with your partner, great! But the time that is likely to be most fertile for finding a compromise will be when she is in the follicular phase. Recognise that you will probably have to give ground if you are going to work together. The real moments of progress are likely to come when there is a natural, open dialogue and an atmosphere of honesty and humility when both partners feel they can admit to being wrong safely. There is nothing more cathartic than mutual confession and reconciliation!

Short-term issues aside, the long-term process of working as a partner with someone with PMDD is one of absolute collaboration. It is the long view that supporting her to improve her health and coping strategies is both a benefit to her and to you. Your destiny is tied in many respects to how successfully the condition is managed.

4. Competition

Someone who uses the conflict resolution strategy of "competition" tries to satisfy their own desires at the expense of the other parties involved. Do you love the thrill of a war zone and like living on the edge? Do you want to make your life as hard as possible? Competing with PMDD is an exercise in futility.

You cannot "break" PMDD; you can only break yourself against it. By all means, try it and see how it goes, but there will be a cost to using this strategy exclusively, and that cost is most likely your relationship. Could your relationship survive that process? This approach has all the hallmarks of a very uncomfortable and traumatic experience. It also does not respect the harrowing experience that someone with PMDD experiences. To prioritise your needs completely and universally over someone else's needs, especially if you are healthy and they are suffering from ill health, is selfishness.

I hope this chapter provided a bit of thought on how you approach conflict and prompted some reflection. It's hardly groundbreaking stuff, but I thought the model was a good framework for viewing your interactions. Above all, it is my opinion that the most important strategy that can be enacted in a PMDD relationship *isn't to defend your position; it's to reinforce your relationship.*

How that reinforcement will be exhibited will likely vary depending on where your partner is in a cycle, but it is to remind both parties as much as possible of the fundamentals of why you exist as a partnership and the ground you have already covered together.

Suicidal Feelings and Actions

From the International Association of Premenstrual Disorders[46]:

"The specific reasons for suicidal thoughts and behaviors are unique to each person. In general, though, suicidal thoughts emerge when emotional distress or pain is high, and an individual feels hopeless (i.e., when someone feels that their emotional distress or pain will never change).

This is especially common in response to stressful events involving other people, such as arguments, breakups, or feeling rejected. These painful experiences often lead people to feel trapped and want to escape, which leads to thoughts about suicide.

In PMDD, of course, emotional distress tends to peak in the luteal phase, when the PMDD brain has an abnormal response to changes in the metabolites of hormones. This abnormal emotional response to normal cycling hormones can be seen in daily emotion ratings but has also been demonstrated in brain imaging studies as well as in brain cells grown from the genetic material of people with PMDD.

So again, these biological sensitivities in the brain lead to feelings of intense emotional distress in the luteal phase, and may also lead to feelings of hopelessness about improving one's situation.

When these factors happen together, particularly when social stressors are involved, suicidal thoughts can emerge. Often in PMDD, these feelings go away after menstruation occurs."

Suicide and Ideation

Research would suggest that those who have PMDD usually have another bonus psychological diagnosis to accompany it e.g. depression, anxiety, bipolar disorder etc.

---

[46] www.IAPMD.org

It can take a long time to get a diagnosis of PMDD and so there is a chance of picking up a 'mis-diagnosis' or two along the way. PMDD seems to come often with extra psychiatric baggage of some other mental health problems. The wonderful Tory[47] and her merry band of PMDD researchers wondered if suicide thoughts and attempts in PMDD were so high because there was such a high rate of *other* psychiatric disorders. They compared a group who were only diagnosed with PMDD versus a group who had PMDD **and** other psychiatric disorders and looked at how they compared.

Suicidal Behaviours	PMDD & Additional Psychiatric disorder	PMDD Only
Ideation	74%	67%
Planning	52%	41%
Intent	45%	34%
Attempt	35%	28%

What do we learn from this?

1. PMDD and suicidal thoughts and attempts are linked
2. There isn't that big of a difference if you have another psychiatric diagnosis versus just PMDD alone
3. Most people with PMDD will have suicidal ideations
4. A *very* significant number will attempt suicide.

Assessing: What Is the Threat Level?

The threat level can vary day to day, hour to hour— you can't predict this. However, you may be able to get a certain idea of where your partner is by listening and talking to her. Whilst suicide can't always be predicted, a

---

[47] Eisenlohr-Moul, T., Divine, M., Schmalenberger, K. *et al.* Prevalence of lifetime self-injurious thoughts and behaviours in a global sample of 599 patients reporting prospectively confirmed diagnosis with premenstrual dysphoric disorder. *BMC Psychiatry* 22, 199 (2022). https://doi.org/10.1186/s12888-022-03851-0

person may be able to express themselves and talk to you about how they are feeling and there are tools to help you facilitate this.

You may get scared about asking your partner if she has thoughts of suicide. You might think it will encourage her to go on and take her own life. But for many people who have survived a suicide attempt, or who have been helped to avoid attempting suicide, the one common thing they share is that someone asked that hard question: "Do you feel suicidal?", or "Have you made any plans to kill yourself?" As hard as it is, if you ask the question, you must be prepared to accept the answer. Don't judge, don't invalidate their feelings- simply be there for them; listen and let them talk.

The following diagram was adapted from The Columbia Protocol, also known as the Columbia-Suicide Severity Rating Scale (C-SSRS). It is helpful as a very basic prompt in assessing suicide risk.

1	2	3	4	5	6	7
No thoughts	Morbid Thoughts	Suicidal Thoughts	Suicidal Thoughts	Suicidal Intent	Suicidal Intent	Suicide attempt
		No *intent* no *plan*	No *intent* No *plan* BUT method	No *plan*, BUT Intent	Intent & plan	
	"I wish I wouldn't wake up" "I wish I was dead"	"I should just kill myself" "I wish I could kill myself"	"I have thought about overdosing, but I'm not going to"	"I think I am going to kill myself, but I am not sure when"	"I am going to do it tomorrow at home"	

The Columbia-Suicide Severity Rating Scale (C-SSRS)[48] supports suicide risk assessment through simple questions that anyone can ask. The answers help you identify whether someone is at risk for suicide, assess the

---

[48] https://cssrs.columbia.edu/the-columbia-scale-c-ssrs/about-the-scale/

severity and immediacy of that risk, and gauge the level of support the person needs. Users of the tool ask people:

- Whether and when they have thought about suicide (ideation)
- What actions they have taken—and when—to prepare for suicide
- Whether and when they attempted suicide or began a suicide attempt that was either interrupted by another person or stopped of their own volition

The Columbia Protocol

SUICIDE IDEATION DEFINITIONS AND PROMPTS	Since Last Contact	
Ask questions that are bold and underlined	YES	NO
Ask Questions 1 and 2		
1) **_Have you wished you were dead or wished you could go to sleep and not wake up?_**		
2) **_Have you actually had any thoughts of killing yourself?_**		
If YES to 2, ask questions 3, 4, 5, and 6. If NO to 2, go directly to question 6		
3) **_Have you been thinking about how you might do this?_** E.g. "_I thought about taking an overdose but I never made a specific plan as to when where or how I would actually do it....and I would never go through with it._"		
4) **_Have you had these thoughts and had some intention of acting on them?_** As opposed to "_I have the thoughts but I definitely will not do anything about them._"		
5) **_Have you started to work out or worked out the details of how to kill yourself and do you intend to carry out this plan?_**		
6) **_Have you done anything, started to do anything, or prepared to do anything to end your life?_** Examples: Collected pills, obtained a gun, gave away valuables, wrote a will or suicide note, took out pills but didn't swallow any, held a gun but changed your mind or it was grabbed from your hand, went to the roof but didn't jump; or actually took pills, tried to shoot yourself, cut yourself, tried to hang yourself, etc.		

If YES to 2, seek behavioural healthcare for further evaluation.

If the answer to 4, 5 or 6 is YES, get immediate help: Call or text 999/911[49] or go to the emergency room. STAY WITH THEM until they can be evaluated.

This scale is useful if someone is **engaged and able to communicate**. But what happens if a concern for the safety of your partner arises after an argument or perhaps you are shut out? Perhaps you are in different places, or you can't visit your partner.

In these situations, you can try and **find someone who they will talk to**— perhaps a close friend or another family member.

If you can't find someone who your partner trusts and you have genuine concerns about their immediate safety, call emergency services.

In the case of suicide prevention, in a crisis it is better to ask forgiveness for calling emergency services than the alternative. Overreaction is safer than underreaction when it comes to management in this situation, but a proportional reaction is preferred.

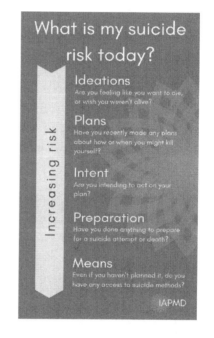

Space Wars

In society there is a continued debate about privacy and security. Two principles that can't seem to get along. Governments want more powers to be able to pry into personal affairs on the premise it is to protect its citizens from terrorism or crime. However, proponents of privacy advocate these powers are unnecessary or invasive. Whether it is CCTV, biometric passports, or detainment laws, they all become a lightning rod for the

---

[49] 988 is the suicide crisis phone number if you are in the USA.

conflict between the principles of privacy and security. This debate not only exists at a societal level, but it works in relationships too, particularly the PMDD relationship.

Your partner sometimes[50] wants space and privacy.
You want to make sure she is safe.

There are numerous times where my partner wanted space or privacy. During acute PMDD it is difficult for someone with PMDD to cope with her own emotions, never mind managing someone else's. Many times, if things had not escalated, I was able to walk away feeling confident that it was safe to do so. Many times, though, I needed to get some space for my own wellbeing.
Sometimes I would be worried about my wife's safety and felt I had to behave like a helicopter, hovering at a distance to ensure that things were OK. I found myself sitting outside a room she might be in, or just sporadically checking in.

Again, if you are sitting on a fence between safety and space, fall on the side of safety. Even better, talk about this prior and build it into your PMDD plan together.

---

50 I say sometimes as at different times, removing myself from a PMDD situation would sometimes be perceived as abandonment or evasiveness. It is a difficult call to make sometimes when your partner is demanding your presence and you feel you need to remove yourself from the situation.

Crisis

During a crisis you might find useful the following CARER guidance by The Carers Trust.[51] This superlative advice can be applied to many other difficult situations.

C – Calm the situation by remaining calm yourself

Check what she is feeling. It's OK to ask, "Are you feeling suicidal?", "Have you made any plans to kill yourself?" or to say, "It's OK to talk to me about how you are feeling."

By asking these questions you are sending out an invitation to let her talk about how she is feeling, or what plans she may have made. You are letting her know you are there for her. People who have experienced suicidal thoughts can find it a relief when someone asks a question about whether they are thinking about suicide, as long as the question is not asked in a judgmental, angry or frightened way. However, don't pressure her to speak. It is OK to ask the question. If your partner doesn't answer, just be with them and don't push too hard.

A – Actively listen

Listen and believe her feelings are very real. Try not to judge her or use guilt or argue with her. If you feel comfortable, and confident to do so, clarify that you have heard her correctly in a calm, neutral tone. Sometimes, when she hears back what she has just said it can make her think and reflect.

Do not try and persuade her that she has a lot to live for or change her mind by pointing out all the good things in life. She is not in any state to be able to see positives, plus you are sending out the message that you are not listening.

---

[51] https://carers.org/caring-for-someone-with-a-mental-health-problem/caring-for-someone-with-a-mental-health-problem

Do not give advice or try to solve her problems.

Don't invade her personal space. Try and give her space and try not to make sudden movements which might panic her. Remember, just by listening you are helping.

R – Reassure your partner that you will stay with them, that you are listening to them

Don't make any judgements, interrogate her or take personal offence. It can be hurtful to hear her think that all is lost and life is not worth living, especially if, as her partner, you have given much time and energy looking out for her. Remember, suicide is not about any other person other than the one with the suicidal thoughts. It is her pain she wants to end.

Reassure her there is help out there. Let her know that most people who have had thoughts of suicide recover and feel better and you will be there during this time.

E – Encourage your partner to seek help

Maybe tell them about helplines they could try or contact their GP for them and encourage them to talk to their GP or a member of the mental health team, if they have one. Let her talk through what issues are present and encourage her to look at alternatives.

If she is drinking alcohol, encourage them to stop; maybe offer her an alternative such as tea, coffee or water. Do not put yourself in danger though by trying to take alcohol away from the person if they don't want to stop.

R – Remember you!

If your partner is in immediate danger of dying, dial 999/911 or (988 in the US) and tell emergency services. Keep yourself safe. If she has a knife or other weapon, do not try and get it from her. Do not give her alcohol or drugs and, if safe to do so, do not leave her alone while waiting for help to arrive. Even if your partner has locked themselves in a room, keep talking to her and keep reassuring her you are there and want to help and listen.

Once the immediate crisis is over, take time to think about yourself. It is not easy to be with someone who is actively suicidal, and it is OK to feel exhausted, angry, upset or scared. These are all very natural feelings but find someone you can talk to about how you feel, whether that be another family member, friend, carer support, other carers or a spiritual person. Find a Carers Trust carer service.

Don't blame yourself—you did the best you could do at a difficult time. If there is no one you can talk to, consider using one of the helplines or write down how you are feeling, listen to some favourite music, go for a walk or just take time out to be kind to yourself. Above all, seek help if you feel it is all becoming too much for you.

Try and remember the word CARER and use the tips above to help.

Additionally, it may be that your partner is able to work through a reflective tool such as the one in Appendix C. It may help your partner disconnect with the suicidal thoughts.

Denying the Cycle

What can you do if your partner doesn't recognise that they have PMDD or does not engage in treatment?

There are two tragedies that I frequently encounter in partner support groups:
1. When a person who is likely to have PMDD won't explore a diagnosis of PMDD and
2. When a partner has been diagnosed with PMDD but refuses to seek treatment.

For partners, these two tragedies can create a very uncomfortable situation. In this chapter, we will look at strategies to enable more engagement with the diagnosis in the hope of improving the situation.

If someone came into your life and gave you a chance to improve it, you'd take it, wouldn't you? Then why, for so many, is there such resistance to either recognising PMDD or seeking treatment? After all, we have established that PMDD can be a massive impairment to a person's life and to those in close proximity. Wouldn't it make sense to try and treat it? Wouldn't you jump on that waggon? While the logic is simple, as usual, *it's a little more complex than that*

Why might a partner with PMDD not seek treatment? Here are a few reasons:
- Fear
- Shame
- Stigma
- Doesn't see the need for intervention
- PMDD makes it hard to seek treatment (your partner will have phases of having less motivation, more negative feelings)
- Sensitivity to hormones may affect memory (oestrogen seems to have powerful role in memory and brain organisation)

- Self-gaslighting from PMDD ("It's not that bad," "My problems are due to other things.")
- She doesn't recognise or acknowledge there is a cyclical pattern
- She doesn't want to know; feels easier to ignore
- Worried about being labelled "crazy," "hysterical" or "broken"
- Worried about losing friends
- Concerned about cost of treatment
- Confidence/low self esteem
- Difficulty talking to medical professionals
- Healthcare access may be limited
- Diagnosis means change/aversion to change
- Previous bad experience with medical professionals.
- Risk of losing employment or other employment related opportunities.

Everyone adapts to the circumstances they are in to a degree. The brain has a degree of plasticity that allows it to adapt to situations, even extreme ones. Many of those who have PMDD may have found themselves normalised to the experience, thinking that "normal" looks like regular cataclysmic arguments on a theatrical scale. *"It's just what happens." "It's just my life."* This process of normalisation is dangerous as it obscures and leaves PMDD issues unaddressed. There is something about being the person with a mental health issue that makes people either hyper-aware of bliss-fully unaware. Mood disorders and anxiety tend to have excessive levels of self-reflection, whilst autism and psychopathy tend to have pathologically low levels.[52] We know there is some sort of link to autism and PMDD, but there hasn't been enough

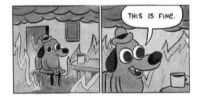

---

[52] Philippi CL, Koenigs M. The neuropsychology of self-reflection in psychiatric illness. J Psychiatr Res. 2014 Jul;54:55-63. doi: 10.1016/j.jpsychires.2014.03.004. Epub 2014 Mar 18. PMID: 24685311; PMCID: PMC4022422.

research to establish what that link looks like.[53]

I spoke to one person who, after 15 years of marriage, confided in a close friend about his home situation. He had thought every relationship was volatile behind closed doors, and only after speaking to a close friend did he realise that it was not "normal," and this eventually led him on a path to discovering his wife had PMDD.

Women who suffer from PMDD may have trouble recognising it too. They have experienced very regular periods of darkness their whole life and may have become desensitised and think the symptoms they have are just "part of life."

The decision to seek or reject a diagnosis or treatment is in their hands. Ultimately, it is *their* body, *their* life, and they are accountable (according to their capacity) and no one else can make that decision for them.

Does this make you powerless to help change the situation as a partner? No.

Does it mean we have to accept there is a limit to what we can do as partners? Yes.
We want to explore and exhaust every ethical avenue to help our partners seek help while still respecting their right to self-determination.

There are two main streets you can walk down with a non-engaged PMDD partner. Either ...

1. Help improve **your partner's** situation – helping your partner to take more *accountability* and *responsibility* (according to their capacity) for getting adequate help for the condition. The success of this is ultimately down to your partner's intention and engagement with the condition and you. Or ...

---

[53] https://faq.iapmd.org/en/articles/7004494-how-many-people-with-pmdd-also-have-adhd-or-autism

2. Improve **your** situation–if your partner won't/can't change–then **you** will have to decide how *you* will improve *your* situation. *Will that be enough?*

If you can improve your partner's life, you will, by default, improve your own. If your partner is not able or won't look for improvements, then what other option do you have but to take control of your own life and your own destiny? It may mean that your decisions are less collaborative and more independent, but just like her, you have the right to self-determination.

Exploring the reasons behind opposition

If you are going to take the first path and help her improve the situation, then understanding the root cause of why she doesn't want to seek treatment is a good starting point. Perhaps you can identify reasons on the list I gave earlier.

Start with the obvious, ask why she is opposed to seeking help (preferably in the follicular phase). It seems basic, but have you *really* asked her? People share their true feelings when they are safe and when someone cares about what they say. Bring a culture of listening into the relationship, ask questions in an earnest, non-threatening way, and compassionately try to understand her world. It takes time to do this–not days, but weeks, months and even years. It takes time and a sustained effort. As an exercise, try to focus only on her point of view. Rephrase and restate back to her what she says to ensure you understand the real meaning of what she says. Do this for a sustained period, and your relationship will improve. Earlier in the book, I talked more about this principle, which is a fundamental relationship building block,

First seek to understand, then seek to be understood.

While you listen to your partner's feelings and points of view, you might not agree, but hold back your instinctual urge to comment or correct. When your partner talks about you or your relationship, you may feel misunderstood, mischaracterized, hurt, and angry. Being able to control your emotions enough to sincerely listen without putting forward your own position is a real challenge. Listening to and understanding your partner in order to help her seek treatment is like brokering peace between warring nations while fighting is still going on. It's going to take time, patience, delicacy, and careful negotiation.

Once you understand the "*whys*," you can start to work on the "*hows*."

Levels of Engagement

If your partner refuses to seek medical care for her condition, then you may feel helpless, redundant, hopeless, immensely frustrated, and angry. Bereft of hope, you may feel consigned to live in an eternal vicious cycle without the ability to escape without ending a relationship with someone you actually love.

You are at the mercy of your partner's decisions, and it can be suffocating. You can't force her to talk. You can't force her to attend appointments with doctors. You can't force her to get the help she needs. You can see a loved one suffering, going through pain and anguish, and it feels like you are a bystander watching a car crash over and over again. Watching the person you love suffer is *agony*. However, there is hope. Whether she knows it or not, if *you* are engaged and helping her seek treatment when she is not, then you are probably her best hope.

The sufferer must be able to access the treatment by engaging with the three Rs.

1. **Recognise** the reality of the condition and the need for help.
2. **Reach out** to competent, relevant medical professionals.
3. **Respond** and engage positively with the advice of medical professionals.

Where is your partner? Is she level 3 or is she level 1? Is your partner just recognising PMDD, or is she actively reaching out and responding to medical professionals? There is no place for undue pressure, excessive coercion, or bullying. While you may be on the receiving end of some unpleasant PMDD symptoms, you cannot replicate the behaviour, as tempting as it might be. Fighting fire with more fire only creates more flames, and everyone gets burned.

Approaching things in an antagonistic way rarely translates into progress during PMDD; it just seems to reduce trust and feeds the paranoid narratives. It seems to exacerbate the unhappiness of the situation and put more blame on you.

There is a phrase I have heard: "How do you eat an elephant?" The answer is "one mouthful at a time." So it is with PMDD. Working with someone with PMDD takes time and lots of small steps. It is the only sustainable way to tackle the medical mammoth that is PMDD.

The first goal shouldn't be for your partner to comprehensively accept her diagnosis of PMDD. The goal should be that she **recognises** that the symptoms she has follows a pattern.

Many PMDD patients have found this "light bulb moment" of recognising PMDD in their lives to be liberating—to know that there is a genuine reason behind their monthly malcontent.

Don't push for total acknowledgement of PMDD in the first instance; recognise that changing minds takes time and needs to be done at the right time. If you look at the diagram below, you can see the different stages your partner may go through in her PMDD recognition journey.

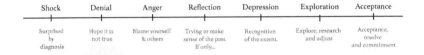

Shock	Denial	Anger	Reflection	Depression	Exploration	Acceptance
Surprised by diagnosis	Hope it is not true	Blame yourself & others	Trying to make sense of the past. If only...	Recognition of the extent.	Explore, research and adjust	Acceptance, resolve and commitment

For some, the diagnosis comes as an *explanation* for so many unpleasant experiences. PMDD may provide an explanation for what was previously misunderstood.

Everyone will respond differently, but models like the one above allow a rough framework to process observations and reflect on what stage your partner is at. Consider also that you are on this journey with your partner, and you will go through these different processes too: shock, disbelief, reflection, but also hopefully exploration and acceptance. The fact that you are reading this far in the book suggests you are probably at the collaboration, exploration, and experimentation stages.[54] It is sad that many PMDD patients report that their partners have never moved on from denial or disbelief.

What can be done to help with non-engagement?

For the rest of the chapter, I will cover some ways you can help your partner become more engaged with the diagnosis. Remember, the aim is to help your partner **Recognise**, **Reach** out for help and **Respond** to professionals' advice.

We are going to cover ...

- Bringing up PMDD for the first time
- Tracking and recording
- Enlisting external help
- Providing audio/video feedback

In the final section of this chapter, I will also provide a summary of options for a partner who doesn't recognise the extent of PMDD and what you can do when you have tried everything and nothing seems to work.

Starting the Conversation

If you are bringing up PMDD with your partner for the first time, it is crucial you do it in the right way. Bringing it up in the heat of an argument

---

[54] Or perhaps it is desperation!

during the luteal phase is possibly the worst way to introduce such a sensitive topic. Consider what TL did in introducing PMDD to his partner. TL is obviously a level 10 PMDD Jedi:

"I had a very calm and delicate conversation about the things we had both noticed about my wife's reactions and I showed her some information that she could read herself I did this while simultaneously making sure she understood that I loved her and that PMDD could be the root cause of a lot of the issues WE were experiencing, and that if she felt that this explained enough, I would continue to support her through this affliction. I also made sure I tried to approach the subject on her good days and did it slowly over a number of months."

Shared on Partner Support, Facebook 2020.

The key principles are all in that statement: calm, delicate, with love and support. I also like the way in which he presents the issue as a *joint problem* to be worked on together and providing her the space and literature to read up on it herself. He didn't affix blame, he didn't rush it, and he offered his support.

There is the chance that, despite your best efforts and considerate delivery, your partner may not respond positively. If discussions don't go well, don't be disheartened. Such a life changing concept can take time to process, and withdrawing from raising the subject for some time may allow space. Concepts like this take time to take root in the mind. They start as a seed, then a green shoot before establishing themselves. Be patient.

Encourage her to track her cycle or read some informative literature.

In the film Inception (*warning: plot spoilers*), a band of mind-hackers, including Leonardo DiCaprio, are tasked with planting an idea in someone's head. The real difficulty, as DiCaprio explains in the film, is that in putting an idea in someone's mind, the person would recognise that the idea had been planted and it wouldn't feel "original" to the thinker. It's true: an idea that feels original to us has more value than someone else's idea. We learn better when we discover something ourselves. It feels more important and authentic when we realise something rather than just being told by someone else. In the movie, they manage to plant the "idea" by sedating the person and creating a dream within a dream. It seemed like an awful lot of effort. Sometimes in the very early days of PMDD, when my wife had not fully recognised the condition she had, I felt like Leonardo DiCaprio in Inception, trying to seed an idea into my wife's mind.

I was trying to ask her to take on my idea of seeking professional help and make it her decision. I knew it had to be her decision, as if she wasn't truly engaged in *asking* for the help, then she wouldn't be engaged in the process of *receiving* the help.

> "Convince a person against their will?
>
> "They are of the same opinion still."
>
> Adapted quote from Mary Wollstonecraft (1759-1797)

Ethical aspects aside, if she was coerced, bullied, or worn down into seeking help, how compliant would she be in trying medication, therapy, or new techniques? What would that do for the trust in the relationship? Self-recognition and motivation are essential. **Your partner has to own the "lightbulb" moment of self -realisation.**

I have been aware of partners who suspected their partner had PMDD and tracked mood changes throughout the cycle then shown the results. The more comprehensive the tracking, the more compelling the evidence will be to your partner. If performed in the right way and in the right spirit of having your partner's interests at heart, it might be something to consider.

This is much preferable to other more extreme ways of presenting evidence. I have known of partners and sufferers secretly recording arguments and replaying them later. I am not sure how great an idea this is! How would you feel if someone was recording you incognito for a couple of months? You wouldn't like it either. This method and other similar tactics are very confrontational, and I would not recommend them unless mutually agreed upon prior.

If there has been a prolonged period where your partner is refusing to seek help and conditions at home are extreme enough, then it might be worth cautiously considering. Something like that would either make or break a relationship.

Delivering any evidence will take sensitivity and certainly should be done at the right time and in the right frame of mind. Relationships are about trust, and to breach that trust is such a big deal. Do the means justify the ends?

One partner I spoke with had success in raising the possibility of PMDD with their partner by highlighting to their partner the physical symptoms that she was experiencing rather than the psychological. Psychological changes are harder to self-identify when you are the person experiencing it. If your partner isn't tracking her cycle, then perhaps you will have to track it and present the evidence.

Have another's help.

When there is a problem in a business, there is value in having someone disconnected from that organisation to come in and solve it. A business consultant or an independent review body are usually commissioned and it allows them to come in and be seen to make decisions objectively. Speaking with business consultants, I learned they feel the recommendations they make can be sometimes obvious, and the large fees they draw aren't because they are saying something groundbreaking, rather objectivity is a commodity that carries a high value. It is the same reason why sometimes people don't take advice from people who are close to them; they worry about conflicts of interest or hidden agendas.

The more objective and authoritative the person is on the subject, the more esteemed their opinion or advice. One of the difficulties of being a partner is that you are VERY close to the situation—you can't be completely objective. Your partner may feel your advice is compromised by your own agenda. To her, your opinion may be biased and one-sided.

This is why you may find that if the ideas come from a source other than you, for example, friends, family, articles or social media, they might be better accepted. It's cleaner, keeping the inter-relationship complexities out of the transaction, leading to a more independent realisation.

Consider, is there a person who might be willing to talk with her? Perhaps there is a medical professional whom your partner already sees and trusts, a friend or a member of the family who is willing to listen and perhaps talk to her. Perhaps they are willing to listen to you and your concerns. If that person understands you are trying to act in the best interests of your partner by getting help, it may work. It is a long shot, and it can be dangerous as anyone who wants to discuss PMDD with her is risking their relationship (and yours!). Unfortunately, I am aware of some with PMDD who only took their mental health seriously when it escalated to the point where partners had to involve the police.

Video/audio feedback technique!

Earlier, I touched on the breach of confidence it would be to secretly record your partner. Whilst I am aware some partners have done this to protect themselves as the relationship descends to a divorce or separation, under normal circumstances I just couldn't subscribe to breaking the trust of someone in that way. I do, however, recognise that extreme situations may necessitate more unconventional methods such as this.

Both people in the relationship need to be able to trust each other, and secret recordings are a massive withdrawal of that trust. Recording someone without their permission may be illegal in some places, but I imagine if someone were experiencing sustained physical or verbal abuse then evidence of that abuse may be necessary if a prosecution were needed. If consent were obtained and the recording were handled in a way that both parties were comfortable with, then I would be comfortable. However, consider the following insightful post by a Reddit user u/scarletunicorn in 2021, reposted with her kind permission. I have included it in its entirety because there is value in every sentence.

"This isn't a happy post, but this is my truth: I'm not sure I have ever really, truly recovered from any PMDD episodes. I literally don't feel like there are enough days in the month between activated and deactivated times to get 'better' so-to-speak. My symptoms subside at the third day of bleeding, and between then and ovulation / the next time symptoms resume, I feel like I barely have the time to catch my breath. If I've had a particularly bad month, I have damaged relationships with people I love very much, and my symptoms subsiding don't undo the damage I have caused. I can't take back hateful things I said when I was enraged and feeling justified, even sanctimonious – righteous in the moment.

"What tends to make me feel better, if anything can, are 1. being productive (personal projects, work goals, that kind of thing) and 2. good times with my boyfriend (I would have said 'family and friends' here but since COVID, I have been pretty quarantined and it's been like a year now, so ... it's just me and him). Still, he has his own messy life throwing challenge after challenge his way, and some of his challenges are just as bad as my PMDD. Some of his challenges are worse. In spite of my best efforts, in spite of who I want to be for him, as my symptoms come back to life each month, my vision narrows until all I really see is me, and how I am being hurt. Attacked. Even if it isn't real.

I recorded us fighting once, because I was so sure he sounded wicked. I'd told him dozens of times that the way he said a thing was not okay. Words matter, but tone does too, and there isn't a human on this planet who would have been okay with the tone he used here or there. 'I love you', said with sarcasm or an exasperated sigh isn't going to make anything better. 'I'm sorry', said flippant and with an eye-roll doesn't make the other party feel seen. I was confident that I was not crazy and if I could play back the recording for him, he too would hear the malice in his voice, the snarky way he said this or that, or that he would recognize that some of his 'requests' were unfair, unreasonable, and often only made to shut me up when I was making a good point. I thought he would apologize at least on a point or two, because my experience is so real to me and I believed what I was hearing. Seeing. Experiencing. Wouldn't anyone?

The recording was frightening. For me. It was like realizing I live in two dimensions. I was there when I was recording him sounding malicious and hateful – my memory was of him being that way – but there on the recording, he was saying the same words and they didn't sound heinous at all. In fact, most of the time, he sounded maddeningly reasonable. He sounded like he was trying to keep it together while under attack ... from me. I sounded how I thought I would sound: outraged, wronged, upset, trying to be heard. That thing he said? That I remembered being so snarky, sarcastic, even angry? On the recording, he sounded ...tired. Just ... tired of it. But in the end, it sounded like he was fighting with me and I was fighting with some totally different version of him that completely eluded the recorder on my phone.

That was a while ago, really, but I still don't know how to recover. I don't know that anyone would know just by looking at me, but I believe my predominant affect is 'haunted'. I am consistently haunted by the awful things I have said and by the awful things that my partner said to me. He's great, but I don't ask or expect perfection from him. He thinks I do, but I don't. Not really. I know everybody has a limit. He screws up too, sometimes – I don't start every disagreement we've ever had. Still, I'm haunted by the questions (should we just call it quits, will this ever get better, what's the point, is everyone better off if I'm alone, did he really mean what he said or did he just say something to hurt me, why would he say it like that, why did I say that hateful thing, why am I like this, will I ever get better, how can I make this right, do they forgive me, do I deserve to be forgiven, how does everyone else manage to live and be productive, why am I so bad at it, etc.) I am haunted knowing I might only feel like 'myself' for a week or two. I am haunted by all of my choices – did I make a life-changing decision because of PMDD or did I really mean it? What is real? Back to the questions, I guess. I am just ... haunted, and it's a cycle I feel really trapped in.

I know what I heard on that recording. I know what I remember, too. I don't know what to do about any of it. I don't know if I can be better. I don't want my relationship to finish falling apart. I keep playing this stupid song in my head:

"'Heart-Shaped Wreckage'"–
Look at this heart-shaped wreckage
What have we done?
We have got scars from battles
Nobody won

If we start over, better
Both of us know
We've got to
Let the broken pieces ...
Let the broken pieces go.

"And I'm in the 'good' part of my cycle right now. These aren't PMDD symptoms; this is me on an asymptomatic day. I want to take a breath, but all I can think of are things like this. The recording. That song. My tattered relationship. My future. Next month has Valentine's Day, and I'm supposed to start bleeding ON the 14th. I'm not doing what I want to be doing. I'm actually living in a situation where I could pursue my ultimate passion project and I'm just ... not doing it. Because I can't relax. I can't take a breath. I feel like I really go through something for a week and a half to two weeks a month, and the rest of the time I spend trying to recuperate, knowing, KNOWING it is all going to start over the moment I get my head above water.
I'm really sad today, you guys. I'm just really sad.

PMDD is so tragic. One cannot help but sympathise with the person who wrote this. For those in a PMDD relationship, it's not just the one to two weeks, it's picking up the pieces for the weeks in between.

It's tragic.

Perhaps you identify with the partner. *"He just sounded ... tired."*

Perhaps you recognise the alternative account of an argument that you both got into. Maybe you have experienced that emotional exhaustion, that psychological fatigue. I thought about how many times I wished my follicular phase wife could be standing beside me with her compassion, sense, and love to carry us both through this moment. I would ache for her return.

I identify with Dani, who has PMDD, and said the following:

"When people ask me what having PMDD feels like, I'd usually respond with the same answer ...

"It feels like grief, like the person you've loved most in the world has died. Complete agony.

"Until it hit me, PMDD does feel like grief, but it isn't mourning the death of someone else. It's mourning the death of yourself. Over and over and over again."

Dani, Posted on IAPMD social media Jan 2022

It was like the person I loved died over and over again, and I would mourn her absence.

I still do not think my wife fully understood how extreme that luteal phase could be in terms of our relationship or the complete change in her behaviour. I would have longed for her to witness the intensity of the experience through another's eyes. Not to add guilt to her pain but to recognise how far she was from herself. Perhaps seeing it from an outside PMDD perspective would have offered more recognition of the demarcation between her and the condition. Perhaps she would have found it easier to forgive herself. Perhaps the process would temper the flames during the next PMDD meltdown.

Video replaying is a brilliant method in sports for improving performance. Perhaps there is a place for both consenting partners to record, critically analyse and evaluate PMDD moments. Would it even help? I am not sure. When talking about this to my wife more recently, she remarked she couldn't have brought herself to listen or watch back if we had recorded a flare-up. It would have crushed her too much. I am not even sure that I would want to relive the experience either. So, I will leave it there.

Summary of options if your partner is refusing treatment or not acknowledging PMDD, and you can't go on.

To summarise, your six options with a non-responsive partner are:

1. *Exist in the current stalemate and hope for something to change organically*

How much damage can you take? How much damage can she take? How much suffering are you willing to tolerate for the relationship to exist? Will things ever change? If life is perpetually miserable, then I suggest that staying in the status quo is not really an option. There is a difference between persistence and obstinance. Persistence is refusing to give up on a difficult goal, whereas obstinance is refusing to consider a different path. Do you need to do something different?

2. *Mission creep: through listening, understanding and empathising*

We have covered a little more previously; strengthening the relationship and opening communication is the preferred foundation of progress and will likely yield the best long-term results. Relationship strengthening takes a long time to do, perhaps even years, and is not necessarily guaranteed to work as it relies on both parties playing their parts. Unfortunately, even with sustained efforts, some relationships may never get to the point where the suffering partner believes in PMDD or the extent to which PMDD affects their life. The self-gaslighting or loss of perspective those with PMDD suffer with can persist, damaging the relationship and preventing access to further care. Despite your best efforts, there is a chance you are still perceived as the source of the problem, not the PMDD. It may also feel more comfortable in living in denial, pretending it's not really happening. For me, however, this method of gentle persuasion worked best for us. It took great energy, time, and sacrifice, with some difficulties along the way.

3. Work with someone she already trusts to help her seek help or recognise the condition

A preference would be to have a medical professional, family member or very close friend who "gets" PMDD and has seen the symptoms firsthand. This person is someone who can listen, who is trusted, and whose opinions are valued. This advocate could help your partner access treatment.

4. Present evidence

Fill out a **symptom tracker** or mood diary for two months and present it as evidence for your partner's consideration. As previously referred to, this method should only be employed if you have exhausted most avenues and is also the highest risk. An intervention like this must be proportionate: you must feel that it is in her best interests and your best interests. Evidence should be presented compassionately, sensitively, and absolutely at the right time.

Number 5 is a heavy one:

5. Ultimatum

I feel a little unsure about writing about this section as it is such a nuclear bomb to a relationship. It never quite got to this stage for me, but I recognise that for some, there might be a situation where it is necessary. Perhaps you as a partner recognise that you cannot cope with the current status quo, or perhaps there are cases where the risk of abuse is sustained and there seems no hope of improvement. Perhaps your partner for a sustained period of time is unwilling to work with their condition. Perhaps your partner does not recognise the extreme impact that PMDD has on their health and wellbeing. Perhaps they do not recognise the essential necessity of engaging in treatment. Perhaps they fail to recognise the impact this has on their partner and immediate family. Perhaps your mental health has become critical. Perhaps boundaries have been broken.

In these situations, the toll can be too much, and the wear and tear of years reaches a threshold, and PMDD threatens to poison the relationship and split the relationship. Let's also recognise that we as partners too can suffer from ill health or addiction, and in that way, our capacity to cope with PMDD may be reduced. I can't imagine having to deal with mental health illness, addiction, or other chronic illnesses while battling PMDD in a relationship. It seems like an insurmountable task.

If your safety is at risk regularly, you have exhausted every other avenue, you have given time for your partner to respond and engage constructively, and you feel you cannot sustain the demands that PMDD has on the relationship and both of you are at the breaking point, then options are very limited.

What options do you have left other than ending the relationship?

Maybe the only option left is an *ultimatum*, e.g., *"Unless you seek proper medical help from a competent medical professional, our relationship cannot continue past x point."*

"Unless we have a plan to improve this situation that we can work together then our relationship cannot continue past x point."

Obviously, you are probably going to have to say a bit more than that. Here is a considered comment by BO from an IAPMD Facebook support group who responded to a post by a partner who was seeking guidance:

"I love you very much, and I don't want our relationship to end, however I can't continue to live this way. I am depressed, losing my identity & can't take the abuse any longer. I just can't. It has become unbearable for me. I am presenting my boundaries & making them clear now in an attempt to not have to end this relationship. If you do not/can not acknowledge the issue & seek out some solutions I will be going my own way in order to preserve myself. I understand

that you are suffering & that it is difficult for you to live with this condition as well, but things can be done to alleviate the pain it's causing you, me & our child. Choosing not to acknowledge the problem & accept the help to minimize the pain we all endure is an admission of disregard for all of our wellbeing. I can't continue in that direction. This is my boundary. I won't honor this relationship with my presence any longer if it is crossed."

BO September 2022

When you make a boundary like this, it is not a threat. What you are laying out are the consequences of inaction. You are explaining what choices you will make. This isn't a request; it's a statement ... a manifesto.

This should not be an off-the-cuff throwaway remark in the heat of a Luteal phase argument; it should be something you have considered carefully and given deep thought and consideration to over a period of months and should be a firm but sensitively delivered message during the non-PMDD phase. It is the iron hand in a cushioned glove. If you can't articulate it in words, write it down in a letter and explain why. Try to emphasise the positives in the relationship, the good things, and make sure that the ultimatum is put in context.

6. *End or reset the relationship.*

Obviously, if all else has failed and the relationship trajectory is one of ongoing destruction, then it may be worth considering ending the relationship. Sometimes things become so broken that they can't be fixed. Ask yourself, "Is this relationship viable?" Are you beneficial to each other? Can the relationship be reset?

Consider the impact on the wellbeing of your partner. It's not her fault that she has PMDD; she doesn't want it any more than you do. Your partner is a prisoner of their own biology and psychology, locked up regularly every month. Your partner has likely endured as much hurt as you have and deserves to be treated with compassion and understanding. The most noble expressions of kindness are displayed during the darkest moments.

My own personal feelings were (and I do not judge anyone who does not walk the same path) that life is complex – you make your decisions, and I make mine. My decision was that I was going to stick this out. For me, my wife, and our relationship, it was worth the pain I went through. I can't help but feel that everything that is worth something in life comes with a price. I paid a high price for what we have today together, but it was worth it. As cliche as it is, I made a promise to be with her in sickness and in health, and I would go through the same again to be where we are now.

Would I have done some things differently? Absolutely!

I'd do it all again, but I would do it better.

It may be worth anticipating and carefully planning how to end the relationship. Does she have support systems in place? Can you talk to a family member or close friend prior or immediately after to help offer that support? If there are children involved, have you anticipated how PMDD may reframe you in the relationship? Falling in love is easy, but untangling two intertwined humans needs a surgical approach; with skill and a delicate hand.

HOPE

Abuse

What I want to make clear from the outset is that no one should be abused; there is no place for it in society, and everybody should have the right to feel safe in their own homes.

I also want to make it clear that just because someone has PMDD, it certainly does not make them an abuser. It would be grossly offensive to the vast majority of PMDD sufferers to make such an ill-considered presumption.

However, I feel this is a topic that is worth examining, not because I want to, but more because it rears its head *very* frequently in partner support. It seems logical to presume that in any relationship where there is more anger, irritability, conflict, and extreme behaviour, there is a higher risk of abuse. Though it is important to point out that there is currently no scientific evidence to suggest that there are higher rates of abuse in PMDD relationships, primarily because there is currently no research being performed on this topic.

Common forms of verbal abuse

Gaslighting - *denying previous incidents took place,*

Blaming - *you are responsible for everything that is wrong*

Shaming - *ridiculing, demeaning behaviour, publicly shaming*

Baiting - *deliberately provoking to become angry*

Name calling - *calling unpleasant names*

It is important to recognise that we all have our own version of what we consider abuse. The Oxford Dictionary gives the definition as *"treat with cruelty or violence, especially regularly or repeatedly."*

Unpicking where abuse lives in the PMDD relationship dynamic is complex and delicate. We know females in general are at a much higher risk of being abused, and we know women who have a history of abuse or trauma are at greater risk of PMS or PMDD.[55] However, it is a chicken and egg scenario—which came first, the trauma or the PMDD? Trauma and PMDD seem to have some sort of bond or relationship, but the relationship seems to be in that awkward "friend zone" stage of not being defined. If you are interested in looking at how trauma may impact physiology and mental health, then you might find this paper by Slavich & Urwin interesting.[56]

The only indicative data available regarding the topic of intimate partner abuse in PMDD is from the survey I took of almost 100 partners of those who suffer from PMDD. The results are shown below:

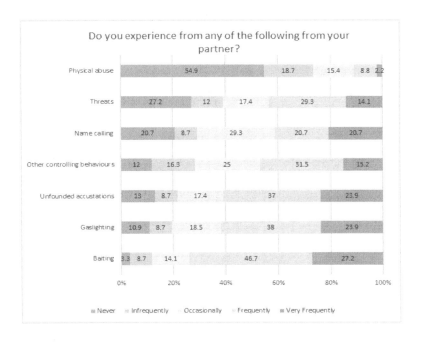

[55] https://faq.iapmd.org/en/articles/2619553-what-is-the-role-of-stress-ptsd-and-or-trauma-in-pmdd

[56] Slavich GM, Irwin MR. From stress to inflammation and major depressive disorder: a social signal transduction theory of depression. Psychol Bull. 2014 May;140(3):774-815. Epub 2014 Jan 13.

- 74% reported experiencing baiting frequently or very frequently

- 61% experienced gas-lighting and unfounded accusations frequently or very frequently

- 45% reported experiencing physical abuse with 10% experiencing the physical abuse very frequently or frequently

I really think abuse in PMDD relationships is a topic that really needs exploring, but I am also wary about the labelling and stigmatisation that already occurs for women. Stories of abuse travel further and quicker in the media than stories of ill-health, pain, suffering and poor support services. I don't want PMDD reduced to a sensational strapline in a tabloid, to become a "condition that makes people abuse their partners". That isn't PMDD.

From my anecdotal experience, the survey results reflected what I expected from conversations and interactions with partners. I am also cautious about talking more about abuse, as I don't feel quite qualified to do so. However, here is some basic advice:

> "Prior to getting my PMDD under control, I was abusive - verbally and physically. I lashed out. I kicked and slapped my partner. He in no way deserved that and I always felt ashamed/suicidal afterwards. Thankfully, I have gotten that aspect under control through therapy and medications"
> PMDD Warrior, PMDD forum

General Advice

- **If you are unsafe, leave the situation.**
  If you can't leave and are unsafe, you can call the police. If you are concerned about the safety of a child or another person, call the police. This applies to short-term scenarios and longer term. If you are unsafe, leave the situation and make a record of what happened.

- **Recognise that abusive behaviour isn't right.** No one should have to live their lives in fear or be unsafe. While during PMDD the sufferer may not have full conscious control during the luteal phase, it is important that they still take responsibility by seeking treatment. Making boundaries for abusive behaviour doesn't mean you don't love your partner.

- Calmly and sensitively **discuss your concerns with your partner** during the follicular phase. In some circumstances, it may be helpful to write down your concerns rather than verbalising them.

- **Get Help.** There are numerous confidential helplines available that offer great advice if you are unsure what to do.

- **Plan for and set boundaries.** Work with your partner where possible to draw up boundaries and a plan. You should plan for what will happen if those boundaries are crossed. If your partner is not engaged in the process or doesn't recognise the behaviour is abusive, it may be necessary for you to plan independently. You have the right to disengage and withdraw if they are being abusive. Setting boundaries means defining where your tolerances lie. It's a preventative act of protection for you and your partner.

- **Keep a record or diary.** While initially this may feel duplicitous, this record can be used to provide evidence of the nature or extent of the abuse. It may help your partner recognise something needs to change. Keeping a diary may also help you recognise the extent of any abuse and the need to take action for your own welfare.

Remember, if your partner's behaviour is abusive and their PMDD is not under control, they are accountable and have the responsibility to seek treatment. If they are not seeking treatment or improvement, it is unlikely the situation will change, and you will continue to be exposed to this type of behaviour. Something must change.

For me there were a particularly terrible few months, I ended up sleeping somewhere else for a few nights, in which time I realised it was emotional abuse. I read through as many of those online check-list things as I could find, and every time I checked more than half of the boxes. I brought it up one time as part of me explaining the new boundaries I would be having and why. I never brought it up as a topic again, but over the next half a year it was brought up by her every month or two, trying to deny, defend, work through it, every time ending fairly badly. I didn't pressure her about it or try to convince her, just stood my ground. Eventually, her therapist talking to her and enough of these conversations has landed us at a point where there has been some acknowledgement and responsibility taken for abuse.

I still think we have a long way to go and things I'd like to talk about given the chance, but my point is that if I had never brought it up or acknowledged it in the first place, and taken a stand and (poorly) set some boundaries, I don't know if she would have taken action for change and we might be in the same or worse place than we were a year and a half ago.

Partner, PMDD forum

4

PLAN FOR PMDD

Plan for PMDD

"In preparing for battle, I have always found that plans are useless, but planning is indispensable."
Dwight D. Eisenhower

One of the great things about PMDD (I think this is the first time I have uttered that phrase) is that, generally, it's cyclical. You know it's going to happen, it's no surprise. Like sailing a battleship out of the harbour on a pushing tide, you can utilise the natural ebb and flow of the ovulatory cycle. The predictability of PMDD reveals a strategic weakness and offers advantage in the war against PMDD:

You know it's coming.

Am I ready for the PMDD luteal phase?

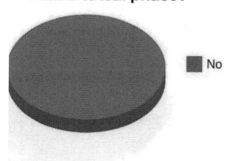

■ No

When I am out surfing, I need to watch out for the bigger waves. They come in "sets," and there can sometimes be up to a 15 or 20 minute gap between these groups of larger waves. Between sets, it is easy to become distracted, normalised by your surroundings, forgetting that these larger waves are looming somewhere over the horizon and that you should be prepared for them. Before you know it, there can be a looming tower of water rolling ominously towards you, and that is the point where there is no time left to reposition or prepare—there is only time to react and scramble past the wave to avoid being destroyed as it explodes into a cascade of whitewater. *You can't stop that wave, but you can position yourself better for it to come.* You can see where I am going with this analogy, right?

In the early days, PMDD would creep up on me from behind like a sneaking massive wave, and I seemed to be perpetually surprised by its resurfacing. Of course, I should have been expecting the onset of the luteal phase, after all, I knew about PMDD. I should have been prepared. It is easy to lose track of how quickly time passes between cycles.

Recording and tracking gave me warning when the Menstrual Gates of Hell were flung open, and it helped me more than I had expected. Eventually, we started sharing a Google calendar together, and we would prospectively add PMDD to the diary so we both knew when it should be hitting. There is an old saying that if you fail to plan, you also plan to fail. I think that is fair. But I also think sometimes the best laid plans can be useless! Ultimately, planning is a way to offset a little of the pain of PMDD, but it is not a panacea—so don't think that just because you have an action plan that it's going to be two weeks of unicorns bathing in fairy dust. Notwithstanding, there are a few different ways you can prepare for PMDD. You have to do your premenstrual PREPS.

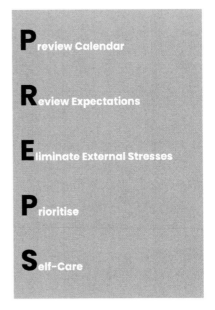

Preview Calendar

Review Expectations

Eliminate External Stresses

Prioritise

Self-Care

PREPS

Preview Calendar

And where possible create a "care plan"

Imagine there was such a thing as a professional PMDD caregiver who came into your home to care for your partner. What would they look like? How would they act? What would they be knowledgeable about? How would they respond in a crisis moment?

When a condition or disease is diagnosed by medical professionals, they will normally produce a "treatment plan" or "care plan," and this plan is then executed by the relevant healthcare professionals. In an ideal world, there would be a trained PMDD care professional who would provide 24-hour care for a PMDD patient according to their needs based on a comprehensive care plan. I imagine if there were a job description for a PMDD caregiver, it might look a little like the following:

Job description: *PMDD caregiver (full time) seven days per week, twenty-four hours per day- but only to a maximum of 2 weeks per month. On call for the rest of the month. No holidays—in fact, you are more likely to have an increased workload during holidays.*

Qualities: *Knowledgeable and trained on PMDD, depression, anxiety, and other adjunctive mental health conditions; able to show boundless empathy. Candidates should be able to provide care under difficult working conditions. You should be comfortable with shifting roles and expectations with little notice. You should be confident in handling a range of mental health crises and confident in providing a range of therapies when needed. Candidates will also be required to undertake a considerable amount of household duties, including cleaning, budgeting, childcare, and not eating too noisily. A range of character qualities will be required, including showing patience, and being unrelentingly* *dependable. The job may involve dealing with difficult scenarios, and only applicants who have high resilience need apply. You may also be called upon to act as a medical advocate.*

As you can see, the bar is set quite high for someone to act as a caregiver for PMDD. Can you imagine having a dedicated professional PMDD care worker in your home? It would be awesome, but they don't exist.

Many a partner didn't realise when they became romantically involved with their partner with PMDD, they also became an inadvertent caregiver. It may not be what they signed up for originally, but ignoring the role of caregiver means ignoring a fundamental aspect of a relationship. The elective decision to take on this role comes as a natural consequence of understanding the health burden your partner suffers from.

Caregiving is a healthy way of providing support and assistance to someone in need - it's motivated by genuine empathy and love. A critical part of being a caregiver is still looking after yourself at the same time. It's a conscious decision to care.

It is not an easy task. Your role and what you can do as a caregiver are best settled with discussion with your partner (in the follicular phase). Points for discussion could be around: "How can I help you deal with this condition?" "What can I learn about PMDD?" and "What can I do better to support you?"

You and your partner should produce a care plan about how you both will try to cope with and make the best of such a life-defining condition. While the majority of the plan is about your partner, a significant portion should be about you too. After all, who cares for the caregivers? Who offers *you* the emotional support during PMDD to get through the hard times? Who understands the difficulties *you* experience? Who can *you* speak to?

How can you make sure the care you provide is sustainable?

The clearer and more upfront we are in talking to our partners about what affects us, the better we can look after each other properly. The alternative is guessing, presuming, and repeating the same mistakes, and everybody feels misunderstood. It is important both parties in the relationship feel comfortable with the plan, which is why it will take a lot of discussion to find the best planned strategies for you both.

Energy accounting

One of the tools that can be used as part of your planning and discussion is "energy accounting."[57] Energy accounting is a method to help you not only understand what is affecting your partner but also the extent to which it affects her. It is a useful exercise in helping to reduce the strain of the luteal phase. The idea is to reduce the damage that PMDD can do.

Energy accounting is not just a method of finding out what is draining, but finding *what is helping or replenishing your partner.* It involves your partner filling out a chart, then sitting down and discussing the findings. The chart should illustrate what events, symptoms, or activities drain energy (withdrawals) and what gives or helps replenish energy (deposits). **The success of the exercise depends on your partner's engagement with the diagnosis. The relationship must be at a sufficient level that these kinds of delicate discussions can be had without escalating into an argument.**

Each item is given a numerical value to give it a weight:
    100 points means it gives/takes a lot of energy
    10 points means it gives/takes a little bit of energy

The idea is that when a withdrawal, or numerous withdrawals, are made, deposits must be made in order to prevent the account from running into overdraft and prevent an acute PMDD meltdown from occurring. Don't be surprised if some of the items on the list seem very mundane or non-events to you; PMDD lowers one's tolerance threshold to make these events an overloading experience.

---

[57] Adapted from the concept of Energy Accounting in autism developed by Dr. Tony Attwood and Maja Toudal

I have created an example below. The **examples and scores given on the list are generic**, and I would expect the list your partner produces to be customised to the specific needs they have.

This is all part of seeking to understand your partner's PMDD, all part of the listening exercise. Review it together and discuss in the follicular phase when both of you feel you are in a good place. Remember, this is a listening exercise with your partner, not an opportunity to share your side (initially).

Withdrawals	Score	Score	Deposits
Criticism/perceived rejection	90	50	Peer support group
Anxiety	70	20	Art
Fatigue	70	40	Having someone else clean
Dealing with doctors	70	40	Sleep
Bloating	20	50	Solitude
Headaches	20	30	Sofa time
Touch	30	30	Reading
Cravings	40	40	Walking
Smells	20	40	Swimming
Being late	50	30	Time with friend
Work pressure	60	20	Music/chosen noise
Childcare	60	30	Foods (specify)
Apathy to interests	60	40	Medication/alt. therapies
Self-deprecating thoughts	70	20	Journaling
Anger	80	20	Mindfulness Exercises
Housework	50	30	Partner doing housework
Crowds/ social gatherings	60	20	Movies/TV
Rejection	70	40	Partner showing kindness by XYZ
Last minute changes	80	20	Yoga

The next step is for **you to perform this exercise**. You, just like your partner, go through the process, noting down the deposits and withdrawals. The two of you should discuss the findings and plan to have dedicated time to share with each other the "withdrawals" and "deposits" and what things you find hard and to what extent.

The findings should then feed into your joint PMDD care plan. A plan should address all the aspects of your life impacted by PMDD. My advice is to shed the stuff you don't need—*simplify your life*. It should not only be what the problems are but, more importantly, *how you are going to deal with them*. Some more ideas and prompts for discussion:

Work arrangements How does your partner deal with work commitments during PMDD? Is there flexibility available from her employer? Can your partner get accommodations? There might be some legal protection for PMDD under discrimination laws. Head to IAPMD.org for more information. Reduction in hours? Working from home? Can she work? Has she had a conversation with the boss? If she is self-employed, do she have good employees and support structures? Do they have income protection insurance? How many days can she take off for illness?

Childcare commitments (primary care responsibilities, feeding, transport) If you have children, how are they being cared for? Is there a way your partner's workload can be reduced? Could you do more in practical terms? Do you have the financial resources to hire extra childcare or help? If your partner needs space, where can you take the kids? Are there locations for short-term stays of a few hours (e.g., the park or the cinema) or even a few days (staying with family)? When your partner is in a bad place, where can you or the children go?

Financial management (budgeting, spending) Debt is frequently a significant stressor. Reducing debt to a manageable monthly amount or clearing it altogether should be high on the plan. Who is going to take care of the finances? Is there an agreement to not make significant purchases during the luteal phase?

"Her Triggers" (a list of potential triggers to be avoided during PMDD)

"Your Triggers" (just as important as "Her Triggers")

Crisis Management (when things get overwhelming and there is a mental health emergency or a meltdown): Who will you call? Local Crisis Team? Police? Family members? Is there a helpline you can call? How can your partner communicate there is a mental health crisis? What do you both define as a crisis? What is the threshold?

Mood-enhancing or distraction activities (what activities help your partner, or at a minimum distract): Exercise? Consider low-concentration activities. e.g., Tetris, Netflix. etc.

Abuse (verbal/physical) What are the red lines that can't be crossed? Where are the boundaries? What are the expectations or agreed consequences if these are crossed?

Food: What foods will be needed? How can the diet be kept reasonable during this time? What binge foods are needed in the home? Is there an easy way to have shopping delivered?

Places and Spaces: How much space does she want? How much space do you need? Live together during PMDD? Live separately during the luteal phase? Is there a room in the house that is more calming, a place where she can go to let it out?

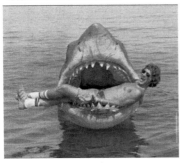

When you and your boyfriend go on vacation but it's also hell week

Holidays and Special Events (Weddings, Family Parties, Work Events, Trips Abroad) There may be unavoidable events (e.g., a wedding, a teacher-parent meeting, a work presentation) that can't be rescheduled. Unfortunately for us, my wife was in the midst of PMDD for our own wedding day and honeymoon. We didn't know at the time, but it tainted the event. My wife is quite candid in saying she didn't particularly enjoy the wedding. PMDD is so cruel; it doesn't respect anything.

Like weddings, there are some events that can't be rescheduled, apologies sent, or cancelled. For those events, there needs to be coping strategies in place. How can your partner practically get through the event without it becoming a meltdown situation? Is there somewhere they can go to take a break from people? Is there a place they can rest if necessary? Is there a way the event could be shortened? Is there a way to partially participate? Does your partner really want to go to begin with?

If your partner is self-aware and engaged in her diagnosis, you can plan together and make a more comprehensive plan. For us, the shared calendar worked, and we would pencil in PMDD, look at upcoming scheduled events, and talk about how we could manage those situations.

If you are at ground zero of engagement with the diagnosis and your partner is in denial, it makes it harder as there will be less collaboration. You may have to work solo on the plan. However, the plan is still important. It enables you to think carefully with a cool head rather than during those intense, emotional times.

Either way, you do the best you can. Put it in your diary, know when it is going to happen, and plan for it.

One important principle to consider when working alongside your partner to produce a plan is that she **has as much autonomy and ownership of her care as possible**. You may find this means taking a step back or supporting decisions that are not what you would do from time to time.

Now that you have it on your calendar and have an outline of some of the subjects in the plan, consider the following principles as you both write up the detail:

Review Expectations

Your partner has a medical condition that renders her capacity reduced for half the month.

It's a disability.

Her life will not be as others live. Your life will not be as others live.

You will have realised by now there are some things that others can do you can't. By accepting the things that you can't change or do alone, you may feel more able to cope. There is some peace with this kind of acceptance. It isn't lowering expectations, it is broadening them.

I feel very averse to any perceived expectation to show affection. My partner is so sweet and affectionate which makes me want to avoid the heck out of him when I'm in this state. Not just physically. Even just having a conversation where he wants to hear about my day or if he shows care or interest in any way it irritates me for some reason, as if it's drama or asking too much. It sounds so mean, but I know I just need to be left alone.

PMDD Warrior, PMDD forum

Consider the following situation: you book tickets for a concert for you and your partner months in advance. You are going to make an event of it, go with a couple friends, get some food, etc. You project in your mind how it's going to be, and you talk with your friends for months about how good it's going to be. As luck will have it, PMDD hits at the wrong time (is there ever a right time for PMDD?), and that concert isn't going to happen the way you thought it was or it's not going to happen at all. The carefree enjoyment turns to tension; nothing about the event sparks joy for your partner. Rather than being bubbly or excitable, the way she was when the tickets were booked, she is now devoid of all happiness. It's like attending a concert while your plus one is at a funeral. You know it's not her fault, but you still feel angry and disappointed. Aren't you allowed to do this one thing that other people do? It feels unfair. Is it too much to ask to be able to go to a concert and enjoy it with someone you love? You look around at the thousands of people in the auditorium and think, "Why me and why her?"

Accepting things are different is hard. You may go through different stages of emotions as you begin to realise the impact of living with PMDD. Your journey through resentment and anger hopefully gives way to feelings of acceptance. Once you have gotten to the point where you accept the reality and can live with it, you can start to customise your life and your partner's life around the condition. However, trying to slot PMDD into a normal, everyday life is like trying to fit an octopus into a tuxedo.

Once *expectations* are adjusted, make reasonable *adaptations*. Using attending a concert as an example, we can show how you might approach planning the event creatively if PMDD strikes:

- Will you attend if PMDD is severe? Perhaps have someone in mind who might want tickets to go to the concert if she can't make it. Be prepared that she may not appreciate your going to the concert without her. Discuss this with her well before booking. Make the decision in the follicular phase. Is she OK with your going to the concert if she is unwell, and who should you go with? Would she/you prefer to both stay at home? Are you able to accept either outcome? How important is this to you and how important is it to her?

- Discuss with the other couples, prior to booking, that there is a chance you may not attend for health reasons. *"Tell me before and it's a reason, tell me after and it's an excuse."* It helps relieve the social pressure your partner will feel, to know there is already an escape route. *"Hey, my partner has PMDD, that means for a week or two every month she suffers very severe symptoms both mental and physical, but mostly mental so it makes planning difficult. We aren't giving excuses as we are really excited and want to go and do this, we are just being realistic about how bad things can get. Unfortunately, we won't know until the day or even the hour if she will be well enough."*

- In the day or two prior to the concert, help your partner get enough rest, eat regularly, take necessary medication, and reduce other random stress factors.

- If she isn't feeling great, could she go for food and drinks before the concert, or meet up after.

- Don't book babysitters at the last moment, arrive with plenty of time, plan your travel well, and have enough cash on you. These are small practical things, but anything that adds to your partner's stress may become a point of conflict or exacerbate symptoms. You know how something small turns into something big.

- Accept that you might do all these things and it might still be an absolute disaster of an evening. C'est la vie.

Sounds like a lot right? It is. But that is the reality of PMDD—the reality of a simple trip blossoming into a cluster of complexity. That complexity makes it difficult to enjoy some of the daily successes, the things that people normally do.

Unfortunately, your Instagram and Facebook feeds are filled with beautiful, shiny, happy people having fun. When you see pictures of people at the concert having the time of their lives, you are at home with your partner in her own private hell. In the words of the Frozen Ice Princess, Elsa, "Let it Go."

When you are at a low point in supporting your partner with PMDD and you are trying to hold it all together, direct yourself to sources of strength or people who are going to support you. There are some Facebook groups for partner support. It is comforting and validating to know others are going through the same thing.

Avoid the temptation to doom scroll through social media. Social media generally only shows you the highlights and the achievements of other people's lives. It's a misrepresentation, as most lives have their own share of drudgery or tragedy. For me, on some days during PMDD, my achievement was "despite attempts by my ill wife to bait me into an argument, I managed to resist and keep my cool." It doesn't make a good Facebook status, though, does it?

By scrolling through media of perfection, we unconsciously start to compare these misrepresentations with our own lives, highlighting the dark place you are in. Tune into your reality, not the social media fables.

Being with your partner, you will have moments of beautiful peace, but you will continue to have heart-wrenching, stomach-churning low points. I recommend psychologically adjusting expectations of what your partner can do physically and productively and how your life is, and you might find those moments of surprise when things just align to produce some wonderful memories.

Eliminate External Stresses (*as much as possible*)

Do you remember earlier in the book when we talked about the HPA axis? This is the body's way of managing stress that lasts for a few minutes. The HPA axis creates a series of events that happen in the body to produce the chemical messenger cortisol. Cortisol is very useful for stressful periods of time. It gives more blood to your skeletal muscles; it increases heart output; and it puts more glucose into your bloodstream. All in all, your body is getting you ready to fight (or flee). However, when these cortisol levels remain high, funny things also happen to the body. For example, the body abandons things that aren't relevant to its *protection*. e.g., reproduction— it's hard to get in the mood for sex while being chased by a hungry bear, right? Priorities change. Chronically raised cortisol has been linked with all sorts of physical and mental health risks; one example is people's immune systems not working properly, leaving them at risk of opportunistic infections. There is evidence the cortisol levels of those with PMDD are affected.[58]

Fight or flight: It is no coincidence that PMDD partners see their loved ones doing one or the other (or both) during the luteal phase. Either your partner is battling you or is trying to leave you. Can you see how this behaviour matches up to a physiological pathway? It is self-preservation; it is warzone thinking. Your partner's own instinctual protective physiology has gotten out of hand.

PMDD exacerbates the real issues your partner faces and inflates them into being so large they are debilitating and suffocating. The bigger the issue is prior to the luteal phase, the more PMDD can wield its devilish incantations

---

[58] Egebladh B, Bannbers E, Moby L, Nyberg S, Bixo M, Bäckström T, Sundström Poromaa I. Allopregnanolone serum concentrations and diurnal cortisol secretion in women with premenstrual dysphoric disorder. Arch Womens Ment Health. 2013 Apr;16(2):131-7. doi: 10.1007/s00737-013-0327-1. Epub 2013 Jan 18. PMID: 23329007.

over it. That work deadline that was mildly stressful is now unmanageable. The coworker who was irritating is now insufferable.

As my wife said *"As my to do list grows, so do my levels of stress. The only way to stop this stress is to get the jobs done. Undone tasks leave me feeling overwhelmed, sometimes so overwhelmed that I can't do any of those tasks.... That's where you come in!"*

We are each like large containers that get filled with stressful things every day. Bit by bit, our volume is filled ... work deadlines, moving houses, changing jobs, debt, relationship issues — ... they all add to filling our containers. You can only take so much before your tolerance threshold is reached and you spill over.

Your capacity to take stress has a limit.

Each person seems to have an inherent capacity. I know people who always seem stressed, no matter what the circumstances. They have a low capacity for stress. For those who have PMDD, their capacity suddenly shrinks, for example, from that of a swimming pool to a bathtub. Things that your partner had the previous capacity to manage are now unmanageable. In this *cortisol mode*, decisions must be made simply and decisively. The nuance and grey areas aren't important when you are being chased by a bear. **It's not that the stresses have changed so much, but the capacity to deal with them has been reduced.**

PMDD reduces your partner's toleration threshold to such a level that it sweeps up everything in life. The non-issues become big issues. Nothing one is exempt: the postman, the cat, politicians, the weather, and a range of inanimate objects can be sources of immense frustration and eternal existential rage. That is why deciding what to eat for takeout on a Friday night can spark World War III.

Even having such a reduced capacity to deal with the stresses is a stress in itself! Such a rapid, steep descent of the onset of the luteal phase does not allow well for adaptive interventions that we would normally take, such as exercise and other self-care methods.

Stress exacerbation during PMDD may make some cycles worse than others. While there may be other physiological reasons for the intensity varying between cycles, stress can make a bad cycle worse. Go through your diary and life and look at things that are going to cause you or your partner stress, the so-called "trigger points". It is important to recognise that there may be things beyond your control (e.g. work commitments, other health conditions, childcare), and some of these you simply can't change, so focus on the things that you can try to improve. You're not superman or superwoman; you can't take on everything, but anything you can do may help just a little.

If it is helping your partner, it is normally helping you.

Moods are contagious in a close relationship. When her capacity threshold is reached, your capacity has also been diminished in the process. You have a limit, and monitoring your own mental health is an important self-care step.

Stress is the pressure or tension exerted on an object. It is often a case of trying to do *too much with too little*—the tasks you undertake with inadequate resources or the emotional burdens without the necessary coping strategies. Managing where we put our resources is a useful way to reduce some stress. Consider for a moment that all the tasks we undertake and the time we spend fit into the following categories: either *urgent* or not, and either *important* or not. This leads us to...

Prioritise

This is a little exercise to review how we spend our time and how we prioritise the most important things. Look at the matrix below.[59]

	Urgent	Non-Urgent
Important	**1** Urgent and Important PMDD acute crisis Deadlines Running out of food or money Family and childcare issues Unavoidable appointments	**2** Non-Urgent and Important Relationship building Medical advocation Research Open discussions Affirming behaviour Exercise and self care
Not important	**3** Urgent and Not Important Interruptions Some phone calls Phone notifications Inexpected visitors Some meetings Some social events	**4** Non-Urgent and Not Important Doom scrolling Junk food Time wasters Some social media Some meetings Destructive behaviours

The time we spend and the tasks we engage in can be allocated into four different categories depending on how urgent or important they are. At different times, we spend more time in each box: e.g. on holiday, it is hoped we spend lots of time doing non-urgent, non-important things, whilst a

---

[59] Based on the Eisenhower Matrix https://asana.com/resources/eisenhower-matrix

visit to the emergency department at the hospital for an acute injury is a classic "urgent and important" scenario.

The matrix above is a good lens through which to view how we spend our time. If you are like me, you might spend an inordinate amount of time dealing with lots of immediate tasks that keep popping up and struggling to get to the important tasks. I often feel like I am firefighting, quickly putting out small fires. Have you ever had an important task to do that you just couldn't get to because of competing unimportant tasks? Are you so busy driving to the places you need to go that you don't get a chance to put air in the tyres or wash the windscreen?

The fourth quadrant of **non-important/non-urgent** is the palace of procrastination—it is the Candy Crush quadrant, Netflix binge watching, doom scrolling on Facebook, or useless work meetings (we "look busy," but the meetings are not very productive. There is nothing wrong with spending a little time here, but time spent here is at the expense of other important or urgent needs. It can prevent you from making meaningful changes in your life and in the life of your partner.

Managing PMDD is all about quadrant two, the **non-urgent/important quadrant,** which I like to think of as the life improvement/life enhancing quadrant. It is here you can plan for PMDD by discussing medical appointments; evaluating the success of interventions; spending quality time with each other when your partner is well; reading positive, helpful things that help you to cope; engaging in refreshing activities that invigorate you and give you the strength to refocus and carry on; or even reading this book! Investing your time here with PMDD is a really good investment, the idea is that you will receive dividends in the long term. Sometimes we spend more time on the urgent tasks because we haven't spent enough preparation time in the non-urgent/important quadrant.

Because of the cyclical basis of PMDD, time is best spent preparing for the luteal phase, where everything kicks off. When PMDD hits, your capacity and motivation will drop, and the preparations you made in the week or two prior to it will feel like a familiar friend coming to help you from the past. We need all the help we can get. We need to be able to hit the ground running.

The luteal phase is the time where crisis management is more likely to occur and you will end up spending more time in the **urgent/important** quadrant. But the preparations you have made will hopefully mean there are fewer distractions and stressors when dealing with the acute symptoms of PMDD.

It is crucial to make your relationship as strong as possible. Dr Alkattan's Doctoral Thesis covers attachment styles and interviews both partners and sufferers of PMDD. It is well worth a read. See the quote from Pearl, interviewed by Dr Alkattan. [60]

"I just feel bad for him, and...I have read a lot of things about PMDD that talk about people wanting to break up with their partners, and, for me, it is more the opposite, that I want my partner to break up with me because I do not want you to have to experience this. I do not want you to have to be around this. I do not want you to see me like this."

Pearl

At times, it seems like you are trying to build a relationship with someone who actively wants to destroy it. It is like swimming against the tide at times, and you wonder if you will make any progress. Patience, persistence, and consistency do normally pay off in the long term.

I recommend re-reading the chapters on building relationships earlier in the book. The better the relationship; the more comprehensive, honest, and effective the plan. If your relationship is at the stage where there is openness and recognition of the condition between you and your partner, you can work collaboratively at a high level in developing a care plan.

---

[60] Alkattan, Rose Anna, "A Phenomenological Study of the Relationship Experiences of Partners of Individuals Who Suffer with Premenstrual Dysphoric Disorder (PMDD)" (2023). *Doctoral Dissertations and Projects*. 4843. https://digitalcommons.liberty.edu/doctoral/4843

Coping During the Luteal Phase:

Don't take it personally.

Yes, easier said than done! Your partner knows you better than most. Your partner knows you intimately, and she knows *exactly* which buttons to press to get certain responses. Your vulnerabilities, triggers, and defences are all mapped out ready to be exploited. Consider this comment made by a partner responding to a Facebook post. The subject of the post was the unkind things that can be said during the luteal phase:

"This all sounds very familiar and it's very difficult to deal with. But it's all the harder if you take what she says to heart. Remember that at these times she feels disconnected from you, desperate and alone. Like her world is falling apart. She will look to blame you for that, but she won't mean everything she says, even if she tells you she means it more than ever. She'll look for any opportunity to criticise (or create opportunities out of nothing) and nothing you do will be good enough. Just do your best to respond with love and she'll remember that when it has passed. But above all, don't take what she says to heart. Being your closest companion, she will know all the best ways to hurt you, and will use them to try and make you feel like she does in that moment. It's so important to distance yourself from the words and try to respond to the pain. I can't emphasise that enough. If you can develop some immunity to the cruelty, it does get (a tiny bit) easier. All the best."

Talking to others about PMDD

In the United Kingdom, it is common courtesy that if you are driving along the road on a motorcycle and you encounter another motorcyclist, you give a little nod with your head. It is an acknowledgement that you are "in the club." It is a way of saying, *"I get you, and I am like you."* Talking to the people involved in your life about PMDD can yield benefits if they are "in the club" and "get it," if they understand what PMDD is.

What is your policy on talking to others about PMDD? I decided when my wife suffered from PMDD that I would only talk to people and inform them of PMDD if my wife had given consent for me to do so. My reasoning was, if I had a condition like PMDD, I wouldn't want my partner telling other people without my permission, because PMDD feels very personal and private, and there is still stigma around mental health issues. I found that naturally, as we came to terms with and worked through PMDD over the years, my wife became more open about it and talked to more people openly about it. As she felt more comfortable talking about her PMDD, I also felt more comfortable talking to others about it.

Looking back now, I feel *sometimes* self-care and getting help can trump confidentiality. People should have a right to share their own life experiences, especially with trusted individuals or therapists. Perhaps I should have talked more to others in the early stages of dealing with PMDD. Perhaps it would have helped me. I think it would have.

It is interesting to see the variability in responses from people when you explain PMDD. Responses may range from non-belief to full acceptance and empathetic understanding; however, having even one other person who really understands PMDD is a massive bonus. PMDD needs understanding, and the wider the circle of support, the easier it can be to live with it.

If, on the other hand, you are dealing with people who 'don't get it' and aren't willing to step outside their own minds, you can feel really alone and isolated.

I am reminded of this PMDD bingo card produced by the amazing Laura Murphy that illustrates what people who "don't get it" might say.

Think positive!	I saw this cure on instagram	Maybe you should exercise	You sleep too much	Do you sleep enough?
Getting surgery for PMS seems a bit extreme	But we all get PMS	PMS can't be THAT bad!?	Have you tried ___?	Are you sure you don't have *insert illness here* instead?
You take too many medications	It could be worse	**PMDD BINGO!**	You can't take time off work for PMS!	Are you better yet?
It's not feminist to say your hormones control you	Have you tried Evening Primrose Oil?	Is that even a real thing?	I get heavy periods too	Why are you crying NOW?!
But you were fine yesterday?	Oh - is it THAT time of the month?	It must be so nice to lay in bed all day	That must be so hard on your partner	VICIOUS CYCLE

Having people around you who understand PMDD helps with the planning and preparation. There may be people you can rely on to help you, either through informal therapy, a place to vent, helping at short notice, or just providing general support. Don't keep it all to yourself; build a team and seek assistance wherever possible. I would recommend that if you don't have someone to talk to, get a therapist so you can work through the experiences you have had to avoid being left with PTSD and a lot of cumulative emotional baggage. IAPMD also offers video support groups for partners, should you wish to attend and have a chat with me!

Lethargy

One of the under-discussed symptoms of PMDD is lethargy and fatigue. Once PMDD hit, my wife would lose all energy. She would become tired and want to sleep more, but even sleeping wouldn't cure her body's insatiable hunger for rest. Along with the lethargy, there was a lack of motivation for life's necessary tasks.

In the absence of having a host of servants and butlers to wait on you and your partner hand and foot, you are probably going to have to pick up the slack during the temporary incapacity. Cleaning, shopping, home repair, paying bills, switching energy providers, organising, events, etc—lots of jobs that are normally shared across the relationship may need to be handled by yourself. I deal with spiders; she deals with tax returns. Between us, running a home with four children is a challenge at times. At one stage in our lives, we had three children under the age of 4, and Jude had cancer. That was an intense time! When my wife was PMDDing, I had to care for her and the children and run the home at the same time. I often felt like an army medic running to and from the next crisis. During PMDD, there was no appreciation or thanks, often quite the opposite, but like the army medic, I did it because I cared for my patient and stepped up to the responsibility.

My wife described experiencing the fatigue as like trying to walk through mud. She said that she felt like her brain was slower, more restricted, and that all energy and any motivation was extracted from her body. I try to imagine what that would make me feel like.

It must be awful to feel lethargy and tiredness for such a prolonged time. Knowing there are things that need doing and experiences to enjoy but not having the energy or capacity to do them is tragic. Many undiagnosed sufferers of PMDD will be thought of as lazy, indolent, or self-serving, while internally they are pleading that this lethargy be removed and productivity and zest for life be resumed.

Like most aspects of PMDD, lethargy has a massive impact on your life as a partner—because you must compensate for your partner's incapacity. It's exhausting working the job of two people. This is why I have such respect and admiration for single parents; they are the diamonds in society, true treasures, and super humans!

It's also very natural not to want to help someone when they are feeling resentful towards you. It's counterintuitive to feel compassion for someone who seems to hate you at that moment. That is why PMDD partners are also absolute solid gold.

There is not much you or she can do about the lethargy during that time. However, both of you can practically prepare for it. I know what I am suggesting is very much "in the ideal world," and practically, it is hard to do. See these further preparations as "pre-premenstrual aspirations." None of the suggestions are ground-breaking, but this list can act as a prompt should you wish to strategically plan.

Further Preparations

Groceries

Try to make sure there is enough food in the house for you and your partner and any other members of the household. You don't want the distraction or additional tasks of multiple visits to the shops.

Distractions

Do you have a Netflix subscription? Binge-watching trash TV is a recognised way of being able to effortlessly continue life for a few hours. Does your partner enjoy a book or a hobby that can act as a distraction during PMDD?

Have an escape route.

I would often worry for my wife's wellbeing when she was home by herself and in the depths of PMDD. Leaving her at home alone in her darkness felt like I was abandoning her; however, you need to still live. In fact, sometimes my leaving the house was exactly what she wanted and what I needed. I understood that at times for her, life was overwhelming, and every single variable was

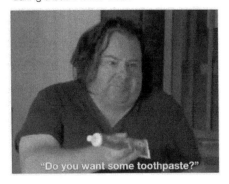

My clueless new partner trying to help me during a bad PMDD week

"Do you want some toothpaste?"

another thing to cause her consternation and anxiety, and having to deal with me was another variable.

As partners, we all need to escape from time to time. Doing something that rejuvenates and replenishes your strength to face life and PMDD is worth it.

For me, it was surfing. I am lucky to live by the sea, and surfing gave me the space I needed. For me, physical exercise and being around nature are both great for mental health.

Premenstrual boundaries.

I cover this a bit more in the abuse section of the book, but it is important clear boundaries are made for what constitutes unreasonable behaviour, which in an ideal world would be agreed upon between partners and discussed *ad nauseum* as part of a care plan. Obviously, this is only possible if your partner is completely on board and engaged in managing PMDD. The boundaries set between you must be fair and proportionate to both parties, and you must be willing to follow through with them. For example, it is critical to decide what

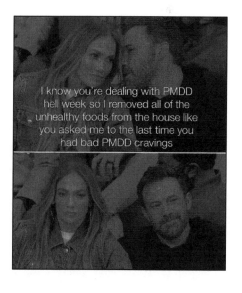

the appropriate course of action would be if your partner became violent or reached the point where suicide is a risk.

Have a well-ordered house.

Before PMDD hits, try to have the house in order. Obviously, it's not going to be high on the priority list, but when everything in your life feels a mess, it can be the only thing that isn't. I always feel a little calmer and like there is more order in my life when my home is in a reasonable state. When PMDD hits, the last thing anyone feels like doing is tidying up.

Childcare

Juggling a crippling, debilitating cyclical condition in the home along with the regular stress of being a parent can be a real challenge. When PMDD hits, what do you do with your children? This is why having other things in order prior to PMDD often means you can focus on the things that matter most. In dark times, my kids were a light (and don't get me wrong, they were hard work) and I honestly felt supported and replensished by their love and that they were "with me" on this journey.

When PMDD hit, the kids and I would often go for a walk or run out to a forest or coast. It would be a break from PMDD for me; I would feel replenished and I would return, I sometimes she would feel a bit better for not having us around. My wife would feel guilty for the lack of proactivity in parenting when she was in the luteal phase. She also found the sensory issues difficult to tolerate, e.g. the noise of having the kids close by in the house. Having the house to herself to sleep in and knowing the kids weren't sitting in front of a screen seemed to lift her mood a small amount. I found many of the efforts I would make weren't life-changing—they didn't alleviate the torture, but I hope they did, in small and simple ways, offset some of the pain of what she was going through.

As always, I felt for my wife, who in normal circumstances would have loved running through fields with us but, through no fault of her own, was unable join us. If you have a family friend, someone who is close, then having the children visit elsewhere may be a good option if PMDD gets really severe or if there is an acute PMDD meltdown. Obviously, if your children are in danger from your spouse, you *must* take appropriate action.

Have a list of activities you can do inside and outside the home. Have enough snacks or food to keep them going. Be realistic in your goals or what you attempt to do with the children; realise that you may feel flat and unmotivated too. Taking them to a local playpark may be more simple and psychologically achievable than some sort of complex, heavily planned, creative, Instagram-worthy craft project.

Help them understand what PMDD is; they deserve explanations as it helps them understand why their parents may behave in a certain way at certain times. I am also aware that for many partners, PMDD really impacts their own mental health, wellbeing, and motivation for life. Trying to look after children, be a source of strength, and "keep it together" seems like an impossible task. If it isn't possible, you need to get help. Sometimes if it was a tough day, I would ask myself, "How can I do this?" "How can I get through this?" The answer would come,

"You have done it before, so you can do it again."

Just one minute, one day, one week, and one month at a time.

Self-Care

"Who supports the supportive partner?" [61]

"Resilience is not resistance to suffering. It's the capacity to bend without breaking. Strength doesn't come from ignoring pain. It stems from knowing that your past self has hurt and your future self will heal.

Fortitude is the presence of resolve, not the absence of hardship."

Adam Grant

Keep It Simple

Self-care doesn't have to involve a whole new life-changing regime and outlook. Your daily regimen doesn't have to be 30 minutes of candlelit yoga listening to Gregorian chants followed by an ice bath and a vegetable smoothie.

A little bit of self-care *consistently*, makes a big difference *ultimately*.

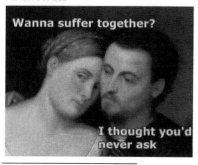

When you find a partner who also has a chronic illness

Wanna suffer together?

I thought you'd never ask

Too many people wait until they're exhausted or depressed to make changes or seek help. Your mental health isn't something you can tuck away, hide or ignore. Make your own "mental hygiene" as regular as "dental hygiene". The daily efforts you make can give sustained rewards.

[61] https://www.buzzfeednews.com/article/chloecaldwell/pmdd-pms-period-related-mood-disorder-searching-for-cure

Find small ways in your day to find some respite. Taking a little exercise, eating healthy food or taking an hour to get some space or switch off can make a difference. Don't drink it away, don't smoke it away, don't eat it away.

Don't think that you can just bulldoze through something like this forever. As you contemplate your experiences, actively take decisions to improve your circumstances. Ignoring your problems just rots you from the inside out.

Get a Totem

I have already mentioned the film *Inception*, in which Leonardo DiCaprio and the other actors can induce a person into a vivid dream. It becomes like a play that other actors in the movie can join in on. The dreams that they conjure are so convincing that the person dreaming thinks that they are real.

You have probably had that experience where you are lost in a dream and it feels so real. The dream world you are living in abruptly comes to an end when you wake up. In the movie, to avoid permanently losing their minds by being psychologically lost in the dream, each of the participants has a 'totem' – an object to help them know if they are in the real world or if they are in a dream. DiCaprio's totem is a small spinning top. The totem acts like a reference point for him, keeping him grounded in what is reality and what is a dream. I often think about this film in the context of PMDD. It seems to have a few PMDD-esque similarities, not the least of which is that DiCaprio's wife suffers from mental health problems, becoming convinced she is in a dream and that in order to "wake up" from the dream she needs to end her life. Despite her husband's earnest pleadings that she is not in a dream world, that she is living in the real world, she misguidedly ends her life.

For PMDD sufferers, the world around them may seem to change so much during the luteal phase – there is disorientation, confusion and false narratives. It must be like living through a bad dream. Understandably It must be hard for those with PMDD to digest that it is not the external world that has changed, but the internal world.

At a recent video support meeting for partners, one of the participants mentioned how they have some pictures on the wall that they use as a reference point to show the happy moments in

> "I used to keep a journal of the arguments, overreactions etc that would happen. I don't anymore, but the first while I did as it helped solidify my emotional well being/mental health. That I wasn't crazy, that I know exactly how/why it went down. I don't read it to her or throw it in her face, it's just there to help me know where I am at."
>
> Partner, PMDD forum

the relationship. This acts as a totem for them. This was going through my mind more recently as I made a photobook for my wife for Christmas. The book contains photos of some of the happy memories we have shared, and I thought about how it might have been a nice gift for her years ago, perhaps it could have acted as a totem for her and for me during the depths of PMDD. In the midst of the hot, sticky mess that PMDD is, I think we all need to be reminded that the possibility of a different, better reality can exist.

Yes, looking at a few photos during a bad time is not going to change anyone's world, but I guess with PMDD, every little effort is worth trying.

Possible Totems:
- Journalling
- 'Memory book'
- Photographs
- meaningful objects
- Visiting a meaningful special/sacred space or place
- Creation of art
- Faith & spiritual beliefs

You both need psychological safe and comfortable places to shelter from PMDD.

Get emotional support.

PMDD can beat you down. Like having a punch to the gut every 10 minutes for two weeks, you get a bit desensitised to the pain, you can get used to it and you resign yourself to things just being "the way things are" and there is "nothing I can do about it". Whilst there may be some things you can't change, there are some things you can.

Often, the biggest obstacle to getting help for ourselves is probably ourselves. The majority of partners are men and it has not been conventionally a "man" thing to do. We tend to just live it out, even when we could do things to make it easier.

I love her with all my heart but I do get very discouraged at times. It is so hard watching the person you love suffer and feeling like you aren't allowed your own suffering because it affects you too.

Partner, PMDD Forum

Support could come from various sources, from friends or family but there are also national carers organisations. In the UK there is an organisation called Carers UK. IAPMD also offers video support groups for partners twice per month and I facilitate one of them. Look up the PMDD partner Facebook groups or the subreddit r/PMDDpartners. These are all places that you can connect with people who share similar lived experiences.

If you're looking after someone with PMDD, regardless of whether you think you fit into any particular definition of a carer, you probably are a carer, and there is support out there. It is just seeking it out. Don't underplay your role.

Be kind to yourself.

When you beat yourself up you don't get stronger or tougher. It just leaves you hurt and diminished. Recognise that you can't heal someone else's PMDD solely through your own behaviour. You aren't responsible for the PMDD. You are not responsible for the anger, depression, or the myriads of other symptoms.

Without doubt, you will have weaknesses, but being kind to yourself isn't about ignoring those weaknesses or pretending they aren't there. Our shortcomings are part of us. Give yourself permission to learn from your mistakes without self-flagellation. Make peace with who you are and what you can do. Look up Acceptance and Commitment Therapy.

Out of my control

The past

The future

The actions
of others

In my control

The opinions
of others

The goals I set

What I give
my energy to

What happens
around me

My thoughts
and actions

The outcome
of my efforts

My boundaries

How I speak
to myself

How I handle
challenges

What other people
think of me

How my partner takes
care of themselves

Understand what you can control and what you can't.

You can't control your partner.

You don't control their words, their actions or their PMDD.

You can control yourself.

You control where your boundaries are.

What goals do you set?

How do you handle challenges and where do you devote your time?

Talk to your employer.

It might seem overkill to talk to your employer, but really, how much does PMDD impact your occupation or performance? In the survey I performed over 50% of partners felt like PMDD had negatively affected their occupation. If you're employed, it might be worth talking to your employer about your situation at home and the responsibilities you have as a caregiver. It can provide some reassurance to have your employer understand that, at different points during a month, you may be under considerable stress. There might be measures they can put in place, such as flexible working, to make sure your work-life balance is manageable.

Maintain your own hobbies and interests.

When you're looking after someone, it's easy to lose sight of your own passions, hobbies, and interests. These are part of your identity – things that make you who you are. The pressures of PMDD may have cut your leisure time down, but it's important to make a little room for these interests. Maintain your identity, who you are, and what you love.

Get enough sleep and eat right.

I emphasised earlier in the book the impact of our physiology on our own mood, and this not only applies to those who suffer with PMDD, it directly applies to us. Sleep and eating healthy are basic tenets of keeping ourselves in the right frame of mind. Are you going to be as caring and tolerant if you have binged on junk food and alcohol and didn't sleep last night? Lack of sleep and not eating right can make stress and depression worse.

Exercise

If you don't exercise regularly, then you are missing an absolute trick. It is hard starting out, but if you find a rhythm or a thing you really enjoy, it can really make a profound difference. When I exercise, I don't feel as lethargic; I feel I have more energy, more hope, and a positive outlook, and it stabilises my mood. When I exercise, it is something I have control over, and it is a personal victory.

When you are dealing with a problem you can't control, like PMDD, the alternative of finding something you can control in your life can be empowering. Walking, weights, cycling, CrossFit, skateboarding, football, rugby, golf ... whatever it is, do it! I found that solitary sports that were easier to slip into a schedule e.g. early morning weight training in the garage.

Other ideas could include mindfulness, journaling, music, yoga, etc. Find something that works for you. One partner made his own "escape tree".

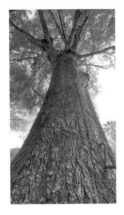

"Today I installed climbing pegs on my oak tree so I can escape. She won't climb a tree. True story. Say hello to my escape tree."
A Partner via PMDD Partners Facebook Group

If you can't cope.

Sometimes the pressure of caring for someone else can build up until it feels like you can't cope. It is nothing to be ashamed of. This is completely understandable, but it is probably a sign that you need to try to rebalance your life toward yourself. If you are feeling desperate and in crisis, you can't keep supporting someone else. You need help.

Conclusion

I hope this book has provided some hope.

I know there will continue to be PMDD-related situations, questions, and circumstances that seem impossible to overcome. I have faith that lives can be improved and changed when couples work together collaboratively and empathetically. This was my experience: a transition from being a victim to becoming a partner sharing the problem—a collaborator, an asset, and an advocate for my wife. Whilst there is no silver bullet for PMDD, it is my belief that no matter what our circumstances, there is always hope.

If PMDD is a poison, then hope is the antidote.

Appendix A: Links to resources:

PMDD Information and Resources

- www.iapmd.org - The International Association of Premenstrual Disorders. A global non-profit organization with a wealth of information and resources on PMDD and PME.

- https://iapmd.org/toolkit - Symptom trackers, care plans and resources.

- Mind Website - UK based mental health charity. One of the few places to have specific advice for family members & partners

- My website - www.pmddhope.com

Video Support Groups

- IAPMD's Partner Support Group is one of several online support groups led by trained peer support facilitators. The group meets once per month and gives the opportunity for partners to share common experiences.
- Click on the following link to find IAPMD's face-to-face peer support meetings ;https://iapmd.org/video-support-groups

Internet Groups

Facebook: PMDD Partner & Families Support Group
https://www.facebook.com/groups/143070706107978
This group only admits partners or family members.

Facebook: PMDD Partner Support Group 2
https://www.facebook.com/groups/1436930706554261
This group admits partners or family members

Reddit: r/PMDDpartners
https://www.reddit.com/r/PMDDpartners
This group admits partners & sufferers of PMDD and is anonymous

Books

https://iapmd.org/other-resources

Additional Resources

Caring Trust

https://carers.org/caring-for-someone-with-a-mental-health-problem/caring-for-someone-with-a-mental-health-problem

Dr Rose Alkattan Psychotherapist has a special interest in the PMDD relationship. https://www.inlovewithpmdd.com/

Appendix B: Partners Survey

A Preliminary Survey into the Impact of Premenstrual Dysphoric Disorder (PMDD) on Partners.

Aaron Kinghorn May 2021

Background

I had the opportunity to witness the severity of the chronic and debilitating condition that PMDD is over a 15-year period and the direct impact on a sufferer's life. I recognise from personal experience the impact of PMDD can be considerable on partners and caregivers but there is little in the way of support networks, resources or research. Online support groups, whilst certainly valuable, can often feel like an echo chamber. It can be difficult to identify if experiences and perceptions raised on such support groups share commonality with other partners and are true representations of living and caring for someone with PMDD.

I created the questionnaire to investigate broadly how partners perceive the impact of PMDD on their lives and to identify common themes. The questionnaire was not based on any previous research, associated with any academic institute or charity and was intended to be a preliminary pilot to assess whether some of the themes relating to PMDD discussed online would emerge in questionnaire data.

I am sensitive to the fact that women suffering with PMDD also suffer from a conflation of other secondary problems including delayed diagnosis and limited treatment options combined with a fundamental ignorance of the condition on a global scale. More awareness, resources and treatment are not simply desirable, they are critically essential and long overdue for PMDD patients. For this reason I am mindful that sufferers stay at the centre of the PMDD experience and that examining the experience of partners does not undermine or detract from the essential work performed to help them.

Partners and caregivers often exist in the shadow cast by their partner's suffering, where the intensity of their partner's PMDD overshadows the difficulties they face. Shining a light on these difficulties will provide dividends for both sufferers and caregivers. Each participant in the PMDD experience deserves to be able to draw out their own space and recount their own lived experiences and views, partners and caregivers included. By supporting and educating caregivers, we provide more of a support framework for sufferers of PMDD. Understanding impact is the first step in a journey to equip and resource the people closest to sufferers to become not simply passive bystanders, but to become educated, supportive advocates who improve the lives of those who suffer whilst synergistically improving their own wellbeing.

Methodology

The inclusion criterion for the survey was set to include only partners of those who had been formally diagnosed with PMDD by a qualified medical professional. Whilst there are many sufferers of PMDD who are undiagnosed or have an informal diagnosis whose partners could have been included in addition to other caregiver groups such as family members or friends, the survey target group was narrowed intentionally to partners of diagnosed sufferers only for specificity. Participants could not undergo the survey unless they had read the introduction-

and the consent section and confirmed they were a partner of someone clinically diagnosed with PMDD.

The survey was anonymous and no identifying data was collected. The survey was conducted using Google Forms and was distributed via social media, primarily on PMDD Facebook groups for both sufferers and partners. The survey ran for one week in March 2021.

Questions were broad-ranging but focused primarily on the partner's perceptions of being in a relationship with someone having PMDD. It touched on topics including the perceived impact on the relationship, physical and mental health, relationships with themselves and others, abuse, mood changes, mental health. Secondary statistical analysis was performed on the results and examined to determine if age, years in the relationship and having a partner undergoing treatment were significant to the results.

Limitations

Participants of the survey may not be representative of all partners. Reach was primarily US/Europe with little participation from elsewhere in the world. Participation in the survey was self-selecting by nature and subject to the limitations inherent to distribution via social media. This method likely excluded partners who did not have access to social media or did not use online support. Additionally, the willingness to participate in the survey may skew the data towards more engaged or affected partners rather than passive or less engaged partners. It may also be that participants in the survey were also a group of partners who struggled more with coping with PMDD in the relationship and; therefore, sought out support groups. There are also limitations in the accuracy of reported perceptions. Perceptions do not always give a true picture of reality. However, in this case because there is no published literature on partners who care for someone who has PMDD, less rigorous evidence such as this can provide a starting point for further well controlled, scientific investigations. There were 96 participants which exceeded expectations, but as always, a higher sample of participants would have been welcomed.
Having no previous experience in conducting research via questionnaire meant questions could have been structured and worded more effectively to gain more constructive and reliable insights. Standardised questions or research tools would have allowed the results to be compared with previous research would have added more rigour.

Demographics of participants

Age

Age distribution was weighted heavily to the 29-49 – year-old range and predictably dropped off around the age when natural menopause would be expected to occur.

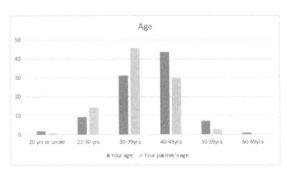

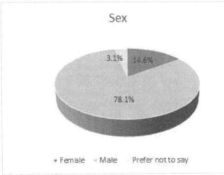

Sex

As expected, the vast majority of partners reported as male (78%), with 15% female. Female same sex couples represent less than 1% in 2019 US census data[1] and this survey shows a much higher representation of same sex couples.

1. htps://www.census.gov/data/tables/time-series/demo/same-sex-couples/ssc-house-characteristics.html

Geography & Religion

- Participants came from US (44%) Europe (41%) and Oceania (8%)
- 66% Identified as no religion and 25% percent identified as Christian

Given the geographic locations of the participants this survey is extremely limited in giving a true global picture. Language barriers, method of distribution of the survey and variable global PMDD awareness could be factors responsible for lack of participation from countries outside the US, Europe and Australia.

Diagnosis of PMDD in the Relationship

At the start of relationships, 66% of participants partners had not been diagnosed with PMDD.
Ten percent of participants were informed of their partner's diagnosis of PMDD at the start of the relationship whilst 20% of partners were not made aware of their partner's diagnosis of PMDD at the start of the relationship.

When asked who first recognised that the participants' partner had PMDD, most partners reported it was the sufferer themselves (51%) with partners recognising PMDD as much as doctors (both reported as 18% by respondents).

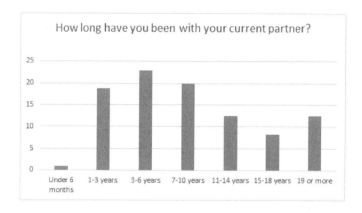

Relationship Duration

The majority of partners had been in a relationship with their current partner for 10 years or less, but generally there was a considerable spread of the length of the relationship amongst partners.

Effect on Life

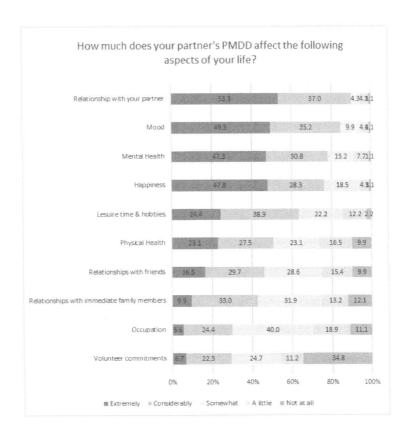

How much does your partner's PMDD affect the following aspects of your life?

	Extremely	Considerably	Somewhat	A little	Not at all
Relationship with your partner	53.3	37.0	4.3	4.3	1.1
Mood	49.5	35.2	9.9	4.4	1.1
Mental Health	47.3	30.8	13.2	7.7	1.1
Happiness	47.8	28.3	18.5	4.3	1.1
Lesuire time & hobbies	24.4	38.9	22.2	12.2	2.2
Physical Health	23.1	27.5	23.1	16.5	9.9
Relationships with friends	16.5	29.7	28.6	15.4	9.9
Relationships with immediate family members	9.9	33.0	31.9	13.2	12.1
Occupation	5.6	24.4	40.0	18.9	11.1
Volunteer commitments	6.7	22.5	24.7	11.2	34.8

90% of partners expressed that PMDD had an "extreme" or "considerable" effect on the relationship with their partner. Between 76% and 85% of partners surveyed described the impact of PMDD on their own mood, mental health and happiness as "extreme|" or "considerable", indicating a notable impact on their general mental wellbeing. The impact was not limited only to the partner's psychological disposition as 50% of participants reported that their partner's PMDD had an "extreme" or "considerable" effect on their own physical health

Whilst not as marked as other factors, PMDD still had a considerable effect on the partners' occupation and relationships with family and friends with 63% of partners reported an "extreme" or "considerable" effect on leisure time or hobbies

Are the Effects of PMDD Positive or Negative?

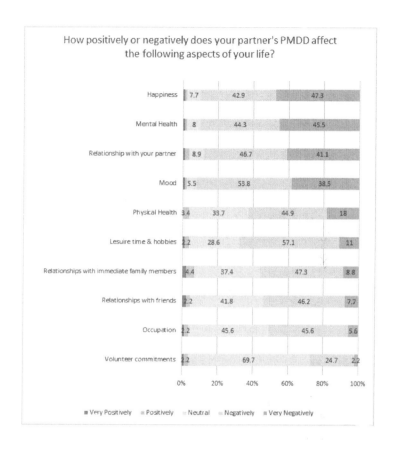

How positively or negatively does your partner's PMDD affect the following aspects of your life?

	Very Positively	Positively	Neutral	Negatively	Very Negatively
Happiness		7.7	42.9	47.3	
Mental Health		8	44.3	45.5	
Relationship with your partner		8.9	46.7	41.1	
Mood		5.5	55.8	38.5	
Physical Health		3.4	33.7	44.9	18
Leisure time & hobbies		2.2	28.6	57.1	11
Relationships with immediate family members		4.4	37.4	47.3	8.8
Relationships with friends		2.2	41.8	46.2	7.7
Occupation		2.2	45.6	45.6	5.6
Volunteer commitments		2.2	69.7	24.7	2.2

Having identified in the previous questions the degree of impact, this question block was used to determine the nature of that impact as being positive or negative. The expectation was PMDD would have a negative influence on aspects of life.

- 92% of partners reported a negative or very negative effect on their own mood
- 90% of partners reported a negative or very negative effect on their own happiness and mental health
- 88% of partners reported a negative or very negative effect on their relationship with their partner
- 50% noted that PMDD had a negative effect on their occupation

Overwhelmingly there was very negative perception from partners on the influence of PMDD on their life with very little positive influence.

Abuse

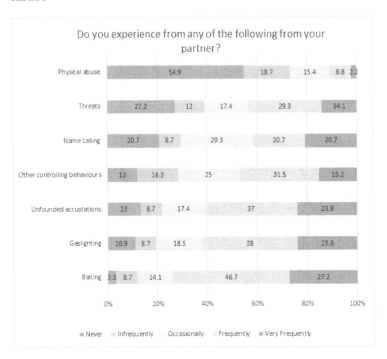

The vast majority of partners reported experiencing some form of abuse.

The most frequent abusive behaviour being baiting. 74% of participants reported experiencing this frequently or very frequently. 61% of partners reported experiencing gaslighting and unfounded accusations frequently or very frequently.

The least frequently experienced form of abuse was physical. However, 45% of partners reported experiencing physical abuse with 10% experiencing the abuse frequently or very frequently.

Despite the high rates of emotional abuse reported in the results of the survey, I urge caution in extrapolation or overstating the results of this particularly emotive topic. Further research with standardised questions and comparative data would be needed to conclude if rates of abuse are prevalent or higher in PMDD relationships.

Stress, Irritability and Mood Changes.

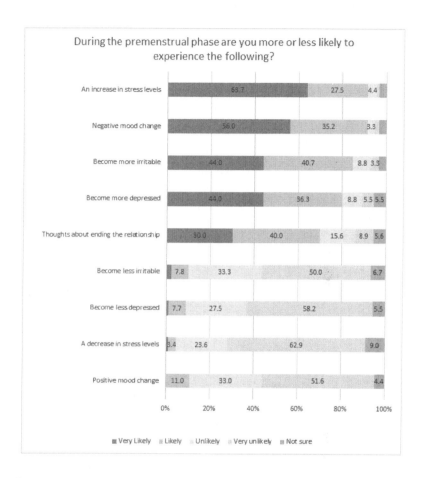

During the premenstrual phase are you more or less likely to experience the following?

	Very Likely	Likely	Unlikely	Very unlikely	Not sure
An increase in stress levels	63.7	27.5			4.4
Negative mood change	56.0	35.2			3.3
Become more irritable	44.0	40.7		8.8	3.3
Become more depressed	44.0	36.3		8.8	5.5 5.5
Thoughts about ending the relationship	30.0	40.0	15.6	8.9	5.6
Become less irritable	7.8	33.3	50.0		6.7
Become less depressed	7.7	27.5	58.2		5.5
A decrease in stress levels	3.4	23.6	62.9		9.0
Positive mood change	11.0	33.0	51.6		4.4

Partners reported they were very likely to experience an increase in stress levels (64%) and negative mood changes (56%). Participants also reported they were very likely to become more irritable and more depressed (44%) during the premenstrual phase.

The majority of respondents confirmed they were very unlikely to experience a positive mood change, a decrease in stress levels or become less depressed or irritable during the premenstrual phase.

The most profound effect seemed to be on stress. 90% of partners reported that they were more likely to experience an increase in stress levels and 89% of partners reported they were less likely to see a decrease in stress levels. 70% of partners reported that they were more likely to have thoughts about ending the relationship during the premenstrual phase

Long Term Impact

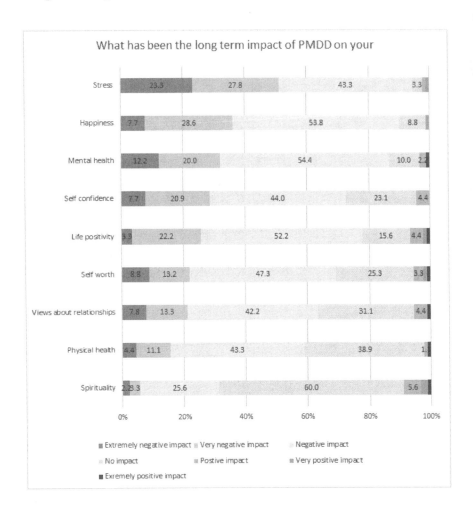

Amongst various factors, participants identified "stress" (94% reported some negative impact) as the factor most associated with having a long-term impact due to PMDD, followed by happiness (90%) and mental health (86%). Individuals' perception of themselves also was negatively affected with 73% reporting a negative effect on self-confidence and 69% on self-worth. 58% reported a negative impact on their physical health.

Perceptions During PMDD

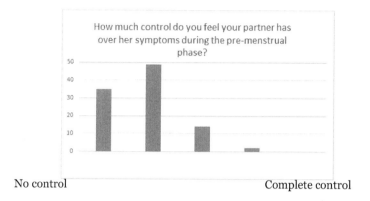

How much control do you feel your partner has over her symptoms during the pre-menstrual phase?

No control   Complete control

Whilst it may seem obvious to many people that there is little to no control over symptoms of PMDD, the questions of control, accountability and responsibility arise frequently on online PMDD groups, and I was interested to ascertain how much control partners felt sufferers had over their symptoms. The majority of partners seemed to recognise their partner had little to no control over PMDD symptoms.

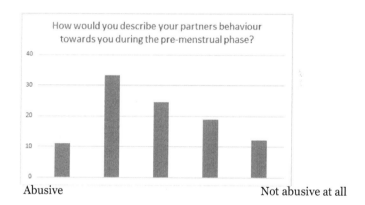

How would you describe your partners behaviour towards you during the pre-menstrual phase?

Abusive   Not abusive at all

Results showed there was a skew towards describing their partners behaviour as abusive during the premenstrual phase. It would have been useful to ask about perceived abusive behaviour during the follicular phase as comparison.

Strength of Relationship

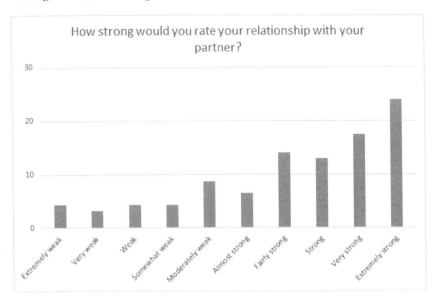

Though the overall picture of PMDD in the relationship was overwhelmingly negative, most participants described their relationship as being strong.

90% of partners felt PMDD had caused them to consider ending their relationship at some stage with 42% reporting that consideration was given very frequently or frequently. This is in stark contrast to the results of the previous question, highlighting the dichotomy of emotions partners feel.

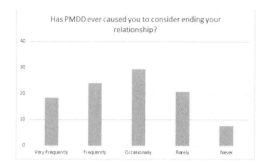

Treatment for PMDD

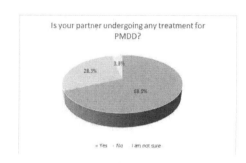

Approximately 28% of participants in the survey reported their partner was not undergoing any treatment for PMDD and 3% couldn't be sure if their partner was undergoing treatment.

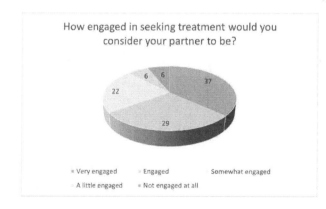

There was a lower participation rate with this question because the question was a continuation from the previous question. Most sufferers who were undergoing treatment were perceived by their partners to be engaged in some way with treatment (87%). However, the significant number of women not receiving any treatment in combination with the number of sufferers not engaging with treatment is of concern and it would be interesting to know if this is representative of the wider population of people diagnosed with PMDD.

Qualitative Questions

What interventions, adjustments or behaviours have you made that have made a positive impact on your partner's PMDD? (optional)
Comments centred around:
Offering emotional support (9)
Not arguing back, not engaging in arguments (7)
Nothing (7)
Giving space (5)
Healthcare advocacy (5)
Offering practical support with routine tasks (3)
Being patient (3)
Tracking cycle (3)

What advice would you give to other people whose partners suffer from PMDD? (optional; 40 responses)

Comments centred around the following themes:

Encourage to seek help and treatments & healthcare advocacy (8)
Be patient and supportive (7)
Understand behaviour is not intentional /-is due to PMDD/is not their fault (7)
Learn about PMDD (6)
Leave relationship (4)
Self-care including avoiding alcohol/drugs(4)
Don't fight, or argue back during PMDD (4)
Be prepared to suffer (3)
Not sure (1)

Statistical Analysis

Analysis of the survey data was undertaken to determine any significant associations between the nature of participants' responses and their ages (<40yrs vs >40yrs), years with partner (<7rs vs 7>yrs) and whether or not the partner's partner was undergoing treatment. Chi-Squared or Mann Whitney tests were applied to the data used to determine if any significant association was found by:

Age

Associations with age were statistically significant (p<0.05) in several areas surveyed. Unsurprisingly, those who were 40 years or older were more likely to have an older partner (p=0.0037 MW) but interestingly seemed to report higher levels of verbal abuse. Respondents over 40 years old were more likely to report name calling (p=0.0216 MW), gas lighting (p=0.0134 MW), controlling behaviours (p=0.0063 MW) and unfounded accusations (p=0.0042 MW).

Older (≥40yrs) partners were more likely to report a negative effect on long term happiness (p=0.0153 MW) but also more likely to describe their partners as having less self-control over symptoms (p=0.0354 MW). The partners over 40 years of age were also more likely to describe their partners as less caring during the premenstrual phase (p=0.0243 MW) and were more likely to report their partners as being less engaged in treatment for PMDD (p=0.0243 MW).

Although not statistically significant, strong associations (p<0.10) were noted that older participants (≥40 years) were more likely to report a negative effect on their physical health (p=0.0786 MW), were more likely to report a negative effect on their relationship with their partner (p=0.0698 MW) and were more likely to report a long-term negative effect on their physical health (p=0.0713 MW).

Older participants were more likely to report an increase in their own irritability during the premenstrual phase (p=0.0690 MW).

Years with partner

Associations with length of relationship (<7yrs vs ≥7yrs) were statistically significant in the following areas. Those who were in a relationship with a PMDD sufferer for 7 or more years were more likely to have an older partner (p=0.0038 MW) and were more likely to report more of an effect of PMDD on their immediate family relationships (p=0.0276 MW). Participants in the relationship for 7 or more years were more likely to report a negative effect on the relationship with their partner (p=0.0212 MW), mental health (p=0.0403 MW) and stress (p=0.0054 MW).

Those partners who had been in the relationship for 7 or more years were also more likely to report their partner as being less engaged in seeking treatment (p=0.0114 MW).

Although not statistically significant, strong associations (p<0.10) were noted in other answers. Participants within a longer relationship (7yrs+) reported PMDD had more of an effect on their happiness (p=0.0866 MW) and on relationships with family members (p=0.0806 MW) as well as being more likely to report unfounded accusations (p=0.0742 MW).

The respondents who had been with their partner for more than 7 years also reported they were more unlikely to experience a positive mood change during the premenstrual phase (p=0.0608 MW) and were more unlikely to feel less depressed during their partner's premenstrual phase (p=0.0860 MW).

The partners who had been in the relationship for 7 or more years reported more of a negative impact on their views about relationships (p=0.0701 MW), and they reported a more negative effect on their life positivity (p=0.0912 MW) and happiness (p=0.0538 MW).

The partners who had been in the relationship for 7 or more years reported they felt their partner had less control over symptoms (p=0.0685 MW) and they felt their partner was less caring during the premenstrual phase (p=0.0723 MW).

Treatment vs Non treatment

The results were examined to assess if there were differences between participants whose partner was undergoing/not undergoing treatment for PMDD. We would expect to see more positive responses in the treatment group. Having a partner who was undergoing treatment was associated with significant differences in several areas, including a less negative impact on the partner's leisure time and hobbies (p=0.0091 MW) and physical health (p=0.0378 MW).

Partners of sufferers of PMDD who were not undergoing treatment were more likely to report experiencing name calling (p=0.0080 MW), other controlling behaviours (p=0.0320 MW) and unfounded accusations (p=0.0375 MW) more frequently.

Partners of sufferers of PMDD who were not undergoing treatment were more likely to report a long-term negative effect on their physical health (p=0.0190 MW) and a long-term negative effect on their views about relationships (p=0.0475 MW). Non-treatment was also associated with impact on thoughts around ending the relationship, where partners who had partners receiving treatment were less likely to frequently consider ending the relationship (p=0.0472 MW).

Other non-significant associations included having a partner undergoing treatment was associated with more positive impact on scores (thought scores were generally negative overall) relating to the long-term impact of PMDD on happiness (p=0.0788 MW), self-worth (p=0.0937 MW), relationships with family members (p=0.0956 MW) and relationships with partner (p=0.0739 MW). An association was observed for how strongly a partner rated the relationship, where those with partners undergoing treatment were more likely to describe the relationship as stronger (p=0.1023 MW).

Key Findings

Diagnosis

PMDD was identified predominantly during the relationship and most cases it was the sufferers themselves who first recognised they may have PMDD. Doctors and partners of sufferers were also groups that first identified that sufferers may have PMDD in almost equal measure, each identifying signs of PMDD first in close to 18% of cases. In 20% of cases the partner was not made aware of their partner's diagnosis at the start of the relationship.

Relationship with Partner

The perceived impact of PMDD on the partner's relationship appears to be significant with 90% of partners in the survey indicating PMDD had an extreme/considerable effect on the relationship with their partner with over half of partners describing the impact of PMDD on the relationship as 'extreme' (53%). Most partners noted the impact of PMDD on the relationship was a negative one (88%). This negativity around their own relationship may help to explain why many partners (63%) felt PMDD had negatively impacted their views about relationships long-term.

Despite the overall negative effect reported by PMDD, most participants viewed the relationship they had with their partner as stronger rather than weaker. Paradoxically, 90% of partners surveyed had considered ending their relationship at some stage due to PMDD with 42% of partners having considered ending the relationship frequently or very frequently. 70% of partners reported they were more likely to consider ending the relationship during the premenstrual phase. Most participants in the survey felt that their partners had no or little control over the symptoms during PMDD.

Mood, Mental Health and Happiness

The survey would suggest partners feel PMDD has a severe impact on their own mood, mental health and happiness. Almost 50% of respondents rated PMDD as having an "extreme" impact on their mood, mental health and happiness.

The nature of the impact was unsurprisingly negative with 90–92% participants describing the impact of PMDD on their mood, mental health and happiness as negative or very negative.

During the premenstrual phase participants reported they were very likely to experience mood changes. Partners reported becoming more irritable and depressed during the premenstrual phase and 90% of partners reported that they were more likely to experience an increase in stress levels during this time. 86% of partners felt PMDD had caused a negative effect on their long-term mental health with 12% describing this impact as extremely negative.

The long-term negative effect of PMDD on a partner's stress and happiness was reported by a very high majority of 94% and 90% respectively.

Abuse

Participants reported they felt they experienced abusive behaviour from their partner. Emotional abuse seemed more prevalent with over 50% of participants reporting they experienced baiting, gaslighting and unfounded accusations on a frequent or very frequent basis. 10% of partners experienced physical abuse frequently or very frequently but conversely 54% had never experienced physical abuse from their partner. From the results of this survey, there would seem to be an association with abuse, the age of the partner and length of relationship.

Physical Health

68% of participants reported a negative effect of their partner's PMDD on their own physical health with 51% of partners describing the impact of PMDD on their physical health as extreme or considerable. 58% of partners perceived PMDD had a negative long-term impact on their physical health. Further research would be useful to know in what ways the physical health of a partner could be affected by their partner's PMDD. Speculation of causes could be around stress, diet, exercise patterns, coping behaviours e.g. addiction and substance abuse.

Relationship with themselves and others

Partners reported PMDD had an overall negative impact on their relationships with friends and family; 17% reporting an extreme effect. Over 50% of partners felt their partners' PMDD had negatively affected their relationships with friends and family members. 50% also felt it had negatively affected their occupation.
Partners also reported a negative long-term impact on their own self confidence and self-worth.

Conclusion

Within the highlighted limitations of the survey, the findings suggest PMDD has a significant negative impact, affecting the stress, the partner relationship and the partners' mental health, mood and happiness. There also seemed to be more negative association with age, length of relationship and having a partner not undergoing treatment for PMDD.

Recommendations

- Given the strong negative perceived impact around PMDD in this survey there is a need for rigorous, peer-reviewed research to explore if these results can be replicated and to examine further some of the themes raised, particularly themes around mental health and abuse.

- Further research is needed to develop evidence-based interventions that could be utilised by carers to improve the wellbeing of sufferers and themselves.

- Establish a formal support network or "space" for caregivers to share best practices and to provide peer support.

Areas to Explore

Given the strong negative perceived impact around PMDD in this survey, a further study could use couples and compare the impact on sufferers and partners as comparative datasets. This would perhaps add more validity to the views expressed if corroborated by both parties in the relationship. Examining exactly how partners currently act as caregivers and being able to identify effective practices may provide valuable actionable recommendations to partners of how to support sufferers. By examining both parties in the relationship, it would also help keep sufferers at the centre of the PMDD dialogue but also highlight the role and impact of caregivers.

Thank you to all partners who contributed to this survey.

Appendix C: Crisis Worksheet

Crisis Worksheet

When thoughts of suicide are overwhelming, staying safe for even 5-10 minutes takes a great deal of strength. This plan is to use during those times. It isn't a plan for how to rid yourself of thoughts of suicide, it looks at staying safe **right now** so you still have the chance to fight another day and access support for whatever is impacting on those thoughts overall. These thoughts and feelings will change, it doesn't mean you will feel like this forever. Let's concentrate on what you can do **right now**.

Why do I want to stay safe?

What are the reasons I don't want to die today? Are there people or animals that make me want to stay safe? Do I have hope that things might change? Am I afraid of dying? Do I want to stay alive just for right now?

....

....

....

....

....

....

Making my environment safer:

Whilst I am focusing on safety, how can I make it harder to act on any plans I might have for suicide? Where can I put things I could use to harm myself so they are harder to get to if I feel overwhelmed?

....

....

....

....

....

....

....

....

....

....

....

....

....

This doesn't mean having to get rid of them forever. It is because I am looking at staying safe right now. If these things make it harder for me to do this, I want to make it harder to use them. This will give me time to connect to that part of me that doesn't want to die.

What might make it harder for me to stay safe right now and what can I do about this?

Do I use any drugs, alcohol or medication to cope? These can make it harder to stay safe if they make me more impulsive or lower my mood. What can I do to make these safe?

....

....

....

....

....

....

....

If I have acted on thoughts of suicide before, what makes it
harder to stay safe that I might need to consider while staying
safe today?

....

....

....

....

Do I have any mental health concerns or symptoms that make it
harder to stay safe? How can I help with these?

....

....

....

....

....

....

....

....

What strengths do I have that I can use to keep myself safe?

What strengths do I have as a person and how might these
strengths keep me safe? What do people who care about me say
about my strengths? Am I creative? Determined? Caring? Do I
have faith or any positive statement I can use for inspiration? How
can I use these answers in my plan to stay safe right now?

....

....

....

....

Who can I reach out to for help?

If I can't stay safe, who is available to help me? Who has helped
me in the past? What helplines or emergency contacts can I use?

....

....

....

....

Long-term support plan:

After staying safe-for-now from suicide, what longer term support
do I want? How might I access this support? What do I need to
change for my thoughts of suicide to change? Where might I start
to get help with this?

....

....

About the Author

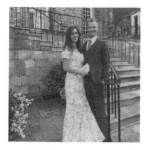 Aaron and Jude live in Durham, England, and have four teenage children. They have been married for 20 years and lived in South Shields, Newcastle and Oxford, before moving to Durham to settle.

Aaron sits on the board of directors for the International Association for Premenstrual Disorders and has hosted a monthly video peer support group for partners for over four years. He was part of the PMDD Community Coalition Roundtable 2021 and presented on the impact of PMDD on partners. He is active in research about PMDD and volunteers alongside Dr Sophie Hodgetts at the University of Durham to try to expand the scientific literature around PMDD, particularly the relationship dynamic.

Outside PMDD, Aaron is chair of the County Durham & Darlington Local Dental Committee and is also chair of South Shields Board Riders Surf Club. He is a volunteer for his church, having served in many different roles over the years.

Aaron loves the outdoors, particularly surfing in the cold North Sea of England.

Instagram:
@mr_the_face
@hopepmdd

Feedback welcome

Dedicated to Jude
I adore you.

Made in the USA
Monee, IL
18 November 2024

70421020R00155